RADICAL REMISSION

Surviving Cancer
Against All Odds

Kelly A. Turner, Ph.D.

HarperOne
An Imprint of HarperCollinsPublishers

HarperOne

RADICAL REMISSION: *Surviving Cancer Against All Odds.* Copyright © 2014 by Kelly A. Turner. All rights reserved. Printed in the United States of America. No part of this book may be used or reproduced in any manner whatsoever without written permission except in the case of brief quotations embodied in critical articles and reviews. For information address HarperCollins Publishers, 10 East 53rd Street, New York, NY 10022.

HarperCollins books may be purchased for educational, business, or sales promotional use. For information please e-mail the Special Markets Department at SPsales@harper collins.com.

HarperCollins website: http://www.harpercollins.com

HarperCollins®, ☕®, and HarperOne™ are
trademarks of HarperCollins Publishers.

FIRST EDITION

Designed by Level C

Library of Congress Cataloging-in-Publication Data
Turner, Kelly A.
Radical remission : surviving cancer against all odds / Kelly A. Turner, Ph.D. —
First edition.
pages cm
Includes bibliographical references and index.
ISBN 978–0–06–226875–4
1. Cancer—Patients—Rehabilitation. 2. Cancer—Psychological aspects.
3. Self-care, Health. I. Title.
RC261.T87 2014
616.99'4—dc23   2013040250

14 15 16 17 18 RRD(H) 10 9 8 7 6 5 4 3 2 1

To all people who have ever heard the words "You have cancer,"
and to their loved ones who have supported them on their journeys.

CONTENTS

INTRODUCTION

anomaly | ə-näm-ə-lē | *noun*: Something that deviates from what is standard, normal, or expected.

You have probably heard a story like this: A person with advanced cancer tries all that conventional medicine has to offer, including chemotherapy and surgery, but nothing works. She is sent home to die but five years later strolls into her doctor's office, healthy and cancer-free.

When I first heard a story like this, I was counseling cancer patients at a large cancer research hospital in San Francisco. During my lunch break, I was reading Dr. Andrew Weil's book *Spontaneous Healing* when I came across a case of what I call Radical Remission. I froze, confused and stunned. Had this actually happened? Did this person really overcome advanced cancer without using conventional medicine? If so, why had it not been on the front page of every newspaper? Even if it had happened only once, it was still an incredible event. After all, this person had somehow stumbled onto a cure for his cancer. The men and women I was counseling would have given anything to know this survivor's secret—and so would I.

Intrigued, I instantly began trying to find other cases of Radical Remission. What I found shocked me. There were over a thousand cases in print, all quietly published in medical journals, and yet here

I was, working at a major cancer research institution, and this was the first time I had ever heard of one.

The more I dug into this topic, the more frustrated I became. It turned out that no one was seriously investigating these cases, nor were they making any attempt to track them. What's worse, most of the Radical Remission survivors I began talking to said that their doctors, while happy for them, often had no interest in hearing about what they had done to get better. The final straw for me, though, was when a few of the radical survivors told me that their doctors had actually asked them not to tell any of the other patients in the waiting room about their amazing recoveries. The reason? So as not to raise "false hope." While it is certainly understandable that these doctors would not want to mislead their patients into thinking another person's healing methods might work for them, it is quite another thing to silence completely these true stories of healing.

A few weeks later, a counseling client of mine broke down in tears while receiving her chemotherapy. She was thirty-one years old, with young toddler twins, and had recently been diagnosed with aggressive stage 3 (out of a possible 4) breast cancer. Through her sobs, she pleaded with me: "What can I do to get better? Just tell me what to do. I'll do *anything*. I don't want my children growing up without a mother." I watched her sitting there, exhausted and bald-headed, with her only hope of recovery dripping slowly into her veins. And then I thought of those thousand-plus cases of incredible, radical recovery, which no one was investigating. Taking a deep breath, I looked into her eyes and said, "I don't know. But I'm going to try to find out for you."

That was the moment I decided to continue on for my Ph.D. and dedicate my life to finding, analyzing, and—yes—*talking about* cases of Radical Remission. After all, if we are trying to "win the war on cancer," doesn't it make sense to talk to those who have already won? In fact, shouldn't we be subjecting these amazing survivors to numerous scientific tests and asking them every question we can think of in an attempt to find out their secrets? Just because we cannot immediately explain why something happened, that does not mean we should ignore it—or worse, tell others to keep quiet about it.

The example I always use is Alexander Fleming, a scientist who chose not to ignore an anomaly. As the story goes, in 1928 Fleming came back from vacation to find mold growing in many of his petri dishes, which was not surprising to him given his long absence. He began sterilizing the dishes, figuring that he simply needed to start his experiment over. Thankfully, though, he decided to pause and take a closer look, and this is when he noticed that all the bacteria in one particular dish were dead. Instead of ignoring this anomalous dish and dismissing it as a fluke, Fleming chose to investigate the matter further—and doing so led him to the discovery of penicillin.

This book shares the results of my ongoing research into the Radical Remission of cancer. It is the outcome of my decision not to ignore these anomalous cases but rather do as Alexander Fleming did: take a closer look. However, I will first give you a bit of my own background, so you can better understand where I am coming from and what inspired me to dedicate my life to this topic.

MY STORY

My experience with cancer began when my uncle was diagnosed with leukemia when I was three. His disease was a long, drawn-out process that lasted five years, casting a shadow over our family gatherings and making all of us young cousins incredibly afraid of that mysterious illness called "cancer." He eventually died when I was eight, leaving my nine-year-old cousin fatherless. That's when I learned that daddies could die of cancer.

A few years later, when I was only fourteen, a close friend of mine was diagnosed with stomach cancer just after our eighth grade graduation. In shock, our small Wisconsin town instantly rallied around him, boosting him up with numerous pancake breakfast fund-raisers and hospital visits. Some of my friends were hopeful, but I could not ignore that feeling of dread deep inside my stomach. After all, I had seen this before. Following two long and side-effect-filled years, my friend died at the age of sixteen. Our entire community attended his funeral, and over the next few years, my other friends and I would go to his grave site regularly to leave flowers. His death taught me that absolutely anyone could die of cancer, at any time.

While earning my undergraduate degree at Harvard University, I was introduced to complementary medicine, yoga, and meditation for the first time. These strange practices and ideas made me start to question my previously held beliefs about the mind and body being separate, and I slowly began to practice yoga. Four wonderful years later, my first job after Harvard was to coauthor a book on global warming, and I suddenly found myself sitting behind a computer all day with none of the social interaction I had enjoyed during college. When a friend suggested that I address my isolation by volunteering, the first idea that popped into my head was to help cancer patients, no doubt because of my early experiences with it.

I still remember my first day volunteering in the pediatric wing at Memorial Sloan-Kettering Cancer Center in New York City. All I did was play Monopoly with some children who were receiving intravenous chemotherapy, but the depth of meaning I felt by helping them forget about their disease for a few hours was truly life-changing. I knew I had found my calling, and after a few more weeks of volunteering, I was already researching graduate school programs. I attended the University of California at Berkeley for my master's degree in oncology social work, with a specialized focus in counseling cancer patients.

While attending graduate school, my interest in complementary medicine deepened, leading me to read many books on the subject and complete an intensive yoga teacher's training course. I spent my days counseling cancer patients and my evenings studying and practicing yoga. At that time, my husband was earning his degree in Traditional Chinese Medicine (acupuncture, herbs, etc.) and also studying an esoteric form of energy healing, so I was surrounded by examples of complementary medicine. It was during this time that I read Andrew Weil's book, which changed the course of my life by introducing me to what Weil calls "spontaneous healing" and convincing me to continue toward my Ph.D., so I could study this fascinating topic in depth. From that point on, I have devoted my life to discovering what people do to overcome cancer against all odds.

WHAT IS RADICAL REMISSION?

In order to understand what Radical Remission is, it is helpful first to think about what is considered "standard" or "non-radical" remission. A doctor expects cancer to go into remission if it is caught early enough and is one of today's more "treatable" cancers. For example, if a woman is diagnosed with stage 1 breast cancer, she will be expected—statistically speaking—to be cancer-free for at least five years, as long as she completes the recommended medical treatment of surgery, chemotherapy, and/or radiation. However, if that same woman is diagnosed with stage 1 pancreatic cancer, there is only a 14 percent chance that she will be alive in five years, even if she completes all the recommended medical treatment.[1] This is because conventional medicine does not currently have treatments for pancreatic cancer that are as effective as those it has for breast cancer.

I define Radical Remission as any cancer remission that is statistically unexpected, and those statistics vary depending on the cancer type, stage, and medical treatment received. To be more specific, a Radical Remission occurs whenever:

- a person's cancer goes away without using any conventional medicine; or

- a cancer patient tries conventional medicine, but the cancer does not go into remission, so he or she switches to alternative methods of healing, which *do* lead to a remission; or

- a cancer patient uses conventional medicine and alternative healing methods at the same time in order to outlive a statistically dire prognosis (i.e., any cancer with a less than 25 percent chance of five-year survival).

Although unexpected remissions are rare, thousands of people have experienced them. I ask all oncologists I meet if they have ever seen a case of Radical Remission in their practice; so far, each one has answered yes. I then ask if they took the time to publish the case, or cases, in an academic journal; so far, each one has answered no. Because of this, we will not know how often Radical Remissions truly happen until we create a systematic way of tracking them. To help accomplish that goal, this book's website—RadicalRemission .com—allows cancer survivors, doctors, healers, and readers like you to submit quickly and easily your cases of Radical Remission, which can then be counted, analyzed, and tracked by researchers. This database is also freely searchable by the general public, so cancer patients and their loved ones can read how other people with similar diagnoses managed to heal against all odds.

ABOUT THIS BOOK

When I first began studying Radical Remission, I was surprised to find that two groups of people had been largely ignored in the thousand-plus cases published in medical journals. The first group was the radical survivors themselves. I found it shocking that the vast majority of academic articles did not mention what the patients thought might have led to their remissions. I read article after article by doctors who carefully listed all the biochemical changes the Radical Remission survivors experienced, but none of the authors reported directly asking the survivors why they thought they had healed. I found this very odd, given the fact that the survivors may have done something—even unwittingly—that helped to heal their cancer. Therefore, for my dissertation research, I decided to find and interview twenty people who had experienced Radical Remission and ask them: "Why do *you* think you healed?"

The second ignored group in the research was the alternative healers. Because most Radical Remissions occur, *by definition,* in the absence of conventional Western medicine, I was surprised no one had studied how non-Western or alternative healers treat cancer. Many of the radical survivors I was hearing about at this time had sought out healers from all corners of the world; therefore, I traveled throughout the globe and interviewed fifty non-Western, alternative healers about their approaches to cancer. I spent ten months tracking down and interviewing alternative cancer healers in the jungles, mountains, and cities of ten different countries, including the United States (Hawaii), China, Japan, New Zealand, Thailand, India, England, Zambia, Zimbabwe, and Brazil. It was a life-changing research trip that led me to meet many fascinating healers, and this book summarizes all that they shared with me.

Since that initial dissertation research, I have continued to find more cases and have now conducted over a hundred direct interviews and analyzed over a thousand written cases of Radical Remission. After analyzing all these cases carefully and repeatedly using qualitative research methods, I identified more than seventy-five different factors that may hypothetically play a role in Radical Remission, including physical, emotional, and spiritual factors. However, when I tabulated the frequency of each factor, I saw that nine of those seventy-five factors kept coming up again and again in almost every interview. In other words, very few of the people I interviewed mentioned, for example, the seventy-third factor, which is taking shark cartilage supplements, but almost every person mentioned doing the same nine things in order to help heal their cancer. These nine key factors for Radical Remission are:

- Radically changing your diet
- Taking control of your health
- Following your intuition
- Using herbs and supplements
- Releasing suppressed emotions
- Increasing positive emotions
- Embracing social support
- Deepening your spiritual connection
- Having strong reasons for living

It is important to note that these are not listed in any kind of ranking order. There is no clear "winner" among these factors.

Rather, all nine were mentioned just as frequently in my interviews, even though—as you will see in this book—some people tended to focus more on one factor than the others. Please keep in mind that the majority of the Radical Remission cancer survivors I study did all nine of these factors, at least to some degree, in their efforts to heal their cancer.

For the sake of organization, I have arranged this book into nine chapters that describe each of these factors in depth. In each chapter, we will first explore the main points of a factor, including taking a look at the latest scientific research on that topic. Then we will explore a complete Radical Remission healing story that highlights that factor. Finally, each chapter concludes with a simple list of action steps that, if you wish, you can take right now in order to start bringing these key factors for Radical Remission into your life.

BEFORE WE BEGIN

Before I share these key healing factors with you, I would like to clarify a few things. First, I would like to state clearly that I am not at all opposed to conventional cancer treatment, including surgery, chemotherapy, and radiation. Just as I believe that most people need shoes to run a marathon, yet a select few have found a way to run twenty-six miles barefoot and healthfully, I similarly believe that most people will need conventional medicine to outrun cancer, while a select few have found ways to overcome it using other means. As a cancer researcher, I am simply dedicated to learning more about the latter group's "training regimen," in an attempt to find out how they achieved such an odds-defying feat.

Second, it is not at all my intention to raise false hope by writing this book. Remember the doctor who did not want his other patients to hear about Radical Remissions? I sympathize with him, because facing a waiting room full of people who have little statistical hope of survival is certainly a daunting task. However, keeping silent about Radical Remission cases has led to something far worse, in my opinion, than false hope: no one is seriously investigating or learning from these cases of remarkable recovery. In my very first research class at UC Berkeley, I learned that it is a researcher's scientific obligation to examine *any* anomalous cases that do not fit into his or her hypothesis. After examining those anomalies, a researcher has only two choices: she can either explain to the public why those strange cases do not fit into her hypothetical model or she can come up with a new hypothesis that includes those cases. Either way, there is absolutely no scenario in which it is okay to ignore cases that do not fit into your hypothesis.

In addition to it being scientifically irresponsible to ignore flat-out the people who have cured their cancers using unconventional means (especially when our shared and common goal is to find a cure for cancer), I would like to discuss the term "false hope." Giving false hope means making people hopeful about something that is untrue or false. Radical Remission cases may not be explainable—at the moment—but they are *true*. These people did cure their cancer in statistically unexpected ways. That is the key difference to understand, so we can get over the fear of raising false hope and begin the process of scientifically examining these cases for potential clues on curing cancer. The nine key factors described in this book are *hypotheses* for why Radical Remission may occur; they are not yet proven facts. Unfortunately, it will take decades of quantitative, randomized trials before we can say for sure whether or not these nine factors definitively improve your chances of surviving cancer.

I did not want to wait decades before sharing these important hypotheses with you. Instead, I wanted to share the results of my qualitative research so we can begin a much-needed discussion about why these cases are being ignored and what they might be able to teach us. The only possibility for raising false hope would be if I were to tell you that you will absolutely cure your cancer if you follow these nine factors. I am not saying that. I am simply saying that, based on my research, these are the nine most common hypotheses for why Radical Remission may occur.

Now that I have made it clear that it is not my intention to raise false hope, let me tell you what I do hope for. First, it is my sincerest hope that other researchers will begin testing these hypotheses for Radical Remission as soon as possible. I also hope that cancer patients and their loved ones will be inspired by this book of true healing stories, just as I was when I discovered my first case of Radical Remission—that they will be comforted by the fact that some people really do recover from cancer against all odds. In addition, I hope this book will motivate people to continue searching for additional ways to optimize their health, whether they are looking to prevent cancer, are in the midst of receiving conventional cancer treatment, or are looking for other options because that treatment has done all it can. Most important, though, I hope this book will be the start of a much-needed discussion about Radical Remissions, so we can stop ignoring them and start learning from them.

———

WHEN IT COMES to cases of Radical Remission, we may not yet be able to understand why these people healed from cancer or why their techniques worked for them but do not always work for others. However, I firmly believe that if we put intense effort into studying these cases—instead of just ignoring them because we cannot explain them—then two possible outcomes will occur: at the very least, we will learn something about the body's ability to heal itself, and at the very most, we will find a cure for cancer. Neither of these outcomes can occur, however, if we continue to ignore cases of Radical Remission. After all, where would we be if Alexander Fleming had ignored the mold in that one petri dish? As history has shown us, studying anomalies is not an unproductive use of time. On the contrary, studying anomalies has historically led to tremendous breakthroughs—and that's where *real* hope lies.

CHAPTER 1

RADICALLY CHANGING YOUR DIET

Let food be thy medicine and medicine be thy food.
—HIPPOCRATES

Hippocrates, the Greek physician who is heralded as the founder of modern medicine, strongly believed that food has the power to adjust, rebalance, and heal the body. Imagine, then, his disappointment if he were to find out that today's M.D.'s receive a total of only *one week* of nutrition education during their four years at medical school.[1] Even at my own recent physical exam, I had to explain to the doctor that, as a vegetarian, I receive plenty of calcium from eating leafy greens (her only suggestion was milk) and plenty of iron from eating beans and seaweed (her only suggestion was red meat). In general, it is not that doctors *disbelieve* in the healing power of food, but rather that they simply never learned about it.

If doctors were to study nutrition in greater depth, they would find that we are indeed what we eat, because the cells of our food get broken down and transformed into the cells of our bodies. In addition, what we eat and drink directly affects our vessels and tissues, making them more or less inflamed depending on what we put into our bodies. To understand this concept, imagine giving a cup of coffee to a five-year-old. After about ten minutes, you would have no doubt that what we eat and drink directly affects our health.

Our health—and indeed our entire lives—can be seen as the sum of all our moment-to-moment decisions. This includes how we choose to eat and drink, think and feel, act and react, and move and rest on any given day. What makes food so powerful is that it is a very *conscious* decision. Will I choose a sugary cereal or oatmeal with fruit? Will it be the quick peanut butter and jelly sandwich or the longer-to-make quinoa salad? For most people, there is a nagging doubt underlying these daily food choices, and it whispers, "Does this really matter? Does what I eat *really* have a vital impact on my health?" The Radical Remission survivors I interview—whose lives are at stake—take that question to the next level. They ask themselves, "Can what I eat help my cancer go into remission?" The answer many of them find is yes.

After analyzing hundreds of Radical Remission cases, one of the nine key factors that consistently comes up over and over again is radically changing one's diet in order to help heal cancer. What's more, the majority of the people I study all tend to make the same four dietary changes. They are:

- greatly reducing or eliminating sugar, meat, dairy, and refined foods,
- greatly increasing vegetable and fruit intake,
- eating organic foods, and
- drinking filtered water.

After discussing each of these changes in depth, I will share two Radical Remission stories from people who radically changed their diets in order to heal their breast and prostate cancer, respectively.

Finally, we will discuss some simple steps you can take in order to start eating an anticancer diet.

NO SWEETS, NO MEAT, NO DAIRY, NO REFINED FOODS

The vast majority of the Radical Remission survivors I continue to research talk about how they reduce or eliminate sweets (sugar), meat, dairy products, and refined foods from their diets in order to help themselves heal. Let's start with sugar. There has been a lot of talk about sugar and cancer, and for good reason. It is an indisputable fact that cancer cells consume (i.e., metabolize) sugar—glucose—at a much faster rate than normal cells do. This is precisely how a PET scan (positron emission tomography) works: first, you drink a glass of glucose, and then the scan detects where that glucose is being metabolized the fastest in your body. Those glucose "hot spots" are the areas in your body that are most likely cancerous. While researchers are still not clear whether a high-sugar diet *causes* cancer, what we do know is that once cancer cells are in your body, they consume anywhere from ten to fifty times more glucose than normal cells do.[2] Therefore, it makes logical sense for cancer patients to cut as much refined sugar from their diets as possible, in order to avoid "feeding" their cancer cells, and instead rely on the glucose found naturally in vegetables and fruits. Knowing that the average American eats the equivalent of twenty-two teaspoons of sugar a day—when we should only eat six to nine teaspoons at most[3]—means there is much room for improvement, whether or not we are currently dealing with cancer.

The connection between cancer cells and sugar was first discovered in the 1920s by a doctor named Otto Warburg. Dr. Warburg won a Nobel Prize for discovering that cancer cells get their energy and breathe (i.e., respirate) differently than healthy cells do. Specifically, he noticed that cancer cells get their energy by breaking down unusually large amounts of glucose and that they also breathe without oxygen (known as "anaerobic" respiration). Healthy cells, on the other hand, break down a much smaller amount of glucose and breathe *with* oxygen (known as "aerobic" respiration). What's interesting is that cancer cells will still breathe anaerobically *even when there is plenty of oxygen around*. This led Dr. Warburg to hypothesize that cancer cells must have something wrong with their mitochondria, since that's the part of the cell where aerobic respiration takes place in healthy cells. Don't worry if you are having anxious flashbacks to high school biology class—the take-home message is simple: cancer cells behave differently than healthy cells do, and one of the key differences is that they require lots of sugar in order to function. Therefore, cutting refined sugars out of your diet may be a key way to help "starve" a cancer cell.

One Radical Remission survivor who changed his diet—and, in particular, cut sugar from his diet—is a man named "Ron." Ron was diagnosed with prostate cancer at the age of fifty-four. His blood tests came back positive for prostate cancer (Gleason score of 6 and PSA level of 5.2), and he tested positive for cancer on two out of twelve biopsy samples. Therefore, his doctors recommended immediate surgery to remove his entire prostate. However, Ron had recently heard of someone who had healed his cancer through nutrition, so Ron wanted first to look into that option. There was no integrative oncologist or nutritionist with whom to talk in his rural town, so he started reading books and articles that explained how cancer cells consume lots of sugar and how many typical American foods, such as white potatoes and white bread, contain it. After a few weeks of intense research, Ron decided to postpone the surgery for a little while and try radically changing his diet instead:

Cancer was probably the best thing that ever happened to me, because I was always pretty keen on fitness, but I did not eat that well. I was a big-time sugar junkie. . . . [To get rid of my cancer,] I eliminated sugar and everything white. No white potatoes, no white bread—that sort of thing. And I ate a lot of greens and did a lot of juicing of cabbage, which I still do, but not as frequently as I could. . . . Cancers are anaerobic . . . and glucose is a nitrogen shuttle, which feeds them. So, if you can just cut off that [glucose] shuttle supply, the cancer is not going to make it.

After changing his diet in this way, Ron's PSA dropped down to a healthy 1.3 in less than a year—and he avoided having his prostate surgically removed, which can have permanent, negative side effects on urinary and sexual function. He has been cancer-free now for more than seven years.

MOVING ON TO dairy products, there are two main reasons that my research subjects suggest that you should reduce or eliminate them from your diet. The first is that dairy is the breast milk of another animal, which means it is packed with hormones and proteins meant to make a baby calf grow—*not* humans. (Incidentally, we are the only species on the planet that drinks the breast milk of another animal.) What's more, research has shown that the main protein in cow's milk, called casein, makes cancer cells grow, both in petri dishes and in lab rats. In fact, researchers have found that they can turn a rat's cancer on or off simply by feeding, or not feeding, it casein.[4]

The second reason that Radical Remission survivors believe you should cut back on dairy is the unhealthy chemicals found in most U.S. dairy products, such as bovine growth hormones, antibiotics, and pesticides. U.S. milk and dairy products have actually been banned in Europe because our cows have been injected with recombinant bovine growth hormone (rBGH), a hormone that has been linked to cancer in various studies.[5] In addition, U.S. dairy products contain unhealthy amounts of omega-6 fats (instead of healthy omega-3 fats), because we feed our cows corn instead of their natural diet of grass[6]—and we only do that because corn is cheaper to grow than grass. The problem with omega-6 fats is they have been consistently linked to cancer.[7]

Finally, it is important to remember that dairy products do not provide us with any nutrients we cannot get elsewhere, even though TV commercials may try to convince us otherwise. For example, we can get just as much calcium from leafy greens and turnips and just as much protein from beans and nuts. Taken together, the evidence is mounting to show that dairy may be cancer promoting, whether due to its inherent casein protein or to the bad things we add to it during production. That is why so many of the radical survivors I study drastically reduce or eliminate their dairy consumption, at least until their cancer is completely gone.

Jane Plant is an example of someone who healed her cancer by focusing on eliminating dairy (among other things). Jane was initially diagnosed with stage 1 breast cancer at the age of forty-two, when her doctors assured her that a mastectomy would "take care of it." Unfortunately, they were wrong. Her cancer recurred a total of five different times, and over the course of the next decade she underwent three additional surgeries, thirty-five radiation treatments, and twelve chemotherapy cycles. When her cancer returned for the fifth time and the latest chemotherapy was having no effect on the egg-size, cancer-filled lymph node bulging out of her neck, her doctors informed her that she had only a few months left to live. As a loving mother and accomplished geologist, however, Jane refused to accept their prognosis. Instead, she began using her skills as a geologist to research what might be at the root of her breast cancer. She had already changed her diet such that she was eating plenty of vegetables and whole grains, but her new research led her to believe there was one additional change she needed to make:

> *In my case, giving up dairy was important. . . . I was having traditional [chemotherapy] treatments at the time, but they weren't working, and it wasn't until I gave up dairy that the treatments started working. . . . I think there are lots of things that cause cancer, but I think you've got to stop the things that promote it, that make it go. . . . It's not as simple as just giving up dairy, though. There are other food and lifestyle changes, too.*

Jane writes about those other changes in her book *Your Life in Your Hands*, which was a bestseller in England. In it, she recommends eliminating all dairy products; greatly increasing one's organic vegetable and fruit intake; eating healthy vegan proteins, such as beans, nuts, and seeds; using healthy oils, herbs, and spices; avoiding refined food products; and drinking filtered, boiled water. She has been cancer-free now for over nineteen years and continues to conduct research on—and stick to—a nondairy, vegetable-rich diet.

———

THE CASE AGAINST meat consumption typically starts with the argument that we humans were designed for a diet that consists of only about 10 percent meat, which ideally should be wild, lean game meat. Today, the average American diet consists of 15 percent meat, which means the average American eats roughly two hundred pounds of meat per year.[8] On the other end of the spectrum, proponents of the Paleo, or "caveman," diet would argue that humans were designed to eat 20 to 40 percent meat. Regardless of what humans were eating thousands of years ago (which is impossible for anyone to prove), at present we are dealing with the modern disease of cancer, and the fact remains that scores of large-scale, well-designed scientific studies have linked regular consumption of meat, especially red meat, to many types of cancer.[9] In fact, one study showed that eating just two servings of meat a day quadrupled a woman's risk of breast cancer recurrence.[10]

In addition to these alarming findings, the meat, poultry, and fish industries have the same issues as the dairy industry when it comes to the unhealthy additives of artificial growth hormones, antibiotics, pesticides, and omega-6 fats. And, as with dairy, there is no nutrient in meat that you cannot get from other sources. For example, vegetarians can get plenty of protein by eating beans along with whole grains and all the iron they need from beans and seaweed. My own conclusion regarding meat consumption is therefore the same as for dairy: if you have cancer, I would recommend drastically reducing or eliminating it from your diet, at least until your cancer fully goes away. If you do choose to eat some meat, make sure it is organic, free-range, hormone- and antibiotic-free, and grass-fed, and limit your intake.

————

THE FINAL FOOD group that Radical Remission survivors reduce or eliminate completely is refined foods, especially refined grains. A refined food product such as bread is made with wheat that has been converted from its original plant form (the fruit of the wheat plant, or wheat berry) and pounded into a fine flour, which is then mixed with yeast and sugar and baked into a loaf. This results in bread that has a very high glycemic index, meaning its carbohydrates are very quickly converted into glucose—which, as we learned earlier, cancer cells love. What's worse is that eating high-glycemic foods, such as bread, pasta, flour, or any quick-cook grain, not only gives cancer cells plenty of glucose to feed on but also creates high insulin levels in your blood, which is yet another condition strongly linked to cancer.[11]

Therefore, in order to keep blood sugar and insulin levels low and stable, the Radical Remission survivors I study drastically reduce the amount of refined foods they eat (or eliminate them entirely) and instead try to eat carbohydrates in their whole forms. Your body digests whole grains much more slowly than refined grains, which helps to keep your blood sugar and insulin levels low. Plus, whole grains have more fiber and vitamins than refined grains do.[12] Perhaps most important, eating whole grains has been consistently linked with lower cancer rates.[13] Examples of whole grains include brown rice, quinoa, whole oats, whole barley, and wheat berries. For bread, you could try sprouted-grain bread, which is denser and has much less sugar per slice than both white and whole-wheat bread.

One of the alternative healers I interviewed is the director of a cleansing program in Thailand, where people from all over the world go to fast and cleanse for three to seven days at a time. To this Thai native, refined foods are so unhealthy that he avoids them completely:

I don't eat fast food, food from a machine, or dairy products. But I eat everything that comes up from nature [i.e., grows in the ground]. That's my daily eating habit. Everything that comes through the can has no life—it's all dead. Think about many factory dates. How does it last for four years? If you pick fruit and chop it, it dies. It lasts three to four days, maybe one day. So, I only eat "alive" food—everything that comes up through nature.

Americans love foods that are made in machines—such as flour and pasta—which are staples of the Standard American Diet (a diet rich in meat and sugars), but it is important to remember that our taste buds do not always know what's best for us. In fact, there is a multibillion-dollar industry dedicated to creating artificial flavors that entice our taste buds so much we cannot help but buy unhealthy, refined food products. Beware also of so-called "natural" flavors, as they are not always what they seem. For instance, did you know that the liquid from the anal gland of a beaver—called castoreum—is often used to create a "natural" raspberry flavor in foods and beverages?[14] It is allowed to be labeled "natural raspberry flavor" by the Food and Drug Administration because it comes from a nonchemical source,[15] but it is certainly not from raspberries.

In addition to enticing us with these artificial and "natural" flavors, processed food companies add extreme quantities of salt, fat, and sugar to most of their products, because they know that our hunter-gatherer taste buds are still programmed to crave these foods, which were in short supply thousands of years ago. Thanks to advances in farming, we can now produce as much salt, fat, and sugar as we want. Unfortunately, evolution has not caught up to this fact, and fast food companies take advantage of that lag. We still salivate like crazy whenever we smell grease (fat), sugar, or salt, which is why it is so hard for us to resist warm french fries.

For all these reasons, it would be wise for cancer patients, or those wishing to prevent cancer, not to trust their taste buds when it comes to making food choices. Instead, the Radical Remission survivors I study return to the lifestyle of their great-grandparents, who ate homegrown vegetables and whole grains, rarely ate expensive delicacies like meat and sugar, and enjoyed significantly lower cancer rates than we do now.[16]

THE HEALING POWER OF VEGETABLES AND FRUITS

When it comes to vegetables and fruits, you already know what I'm going to say: they are healthy for you—*very* healthy. Vegetables and fruits provide the human body with everything it needs: vitamins, minerals, carbohydrates, fiber, glucose, protein, and even healthy fats. In terms of cancer, hundreds upon hundreds of studies have shown that eating vegetables and fruits helps prevent you from getting cancer in the first place,[17] while other continuing studies show that cancer patients who eat more vegetables and fruits live longer.[18] For example, one study that followed fifteen hundred breast cancer survivors found that those women who ate five servings of fruits and/or vegetables a day and were also physically active for at least thirty minutes a day, six days a week had a *50 percent reduction* in mortality compared to those who did not eat as many vegetables or exercise as much.[19] In other words, the cancer survivors who ate lots of vegetables and exercised regularly lived twice as long.

There have also been many studies showing that specific fruits and vegetables are potent cancer-fighters—such as cruciferous vegetables (e.g., cabbage, broccoli, cauliflower), allium vegetables (e.g., onions, garlic, scallions), and dark berries. Cruciferous vegetables alone contain nutrients that help block the growth of cancer cells,[20] stop cancer cells from becoming metastatic,[21] and even make cancer cells pop or die.[22] Meanwhile, other vegetables and fruits have different anticancer properties. Therefore, in order to benefit from all the cancer-fighting nutrients out there, you should try to eat all the colors of the rainbow with your fruits and vegetables, since each color represents a different cancer-fighting nutrient.

One of the Radical Remission survivors I interviewed who discovered the healing power of vegetables and fruits was Dale Figtree. At the young age of twenty-seven, Dale was diagnosed with non-Hodgkin's lymphoma, or cancer of the lymph system. During exploratory surgery, a grapefruit-size lymphatic tumor was discovered attached to her lung, heart, and main arteries, which meant it was inoperable. Dale immediately started chemo and radiation, per her doctor's orders, but was forced to stop the chemo two months later due to severe side effects. After three more months of radiation only, she had to stop that too, because it started to affect her speech. Left with no other options, she started experimenting with a wide variety of body-mind-spirit treatments, one of which was nutrition:

> I went to see a master nutritionist who put me on a food program of all high-nutrient, easy-to-digest foods, with quantities that were huge! It took a few weeks for my stomach to be able to hold that much food, but once it did, I was like a sponge slurping food up. The program was about 80 percent raw food, 20 percent cooked. I had three freshly made vegetable juices daily with huge amounts of salads, fruits, and nuts. At dinner, I had the addition of one pound of cooked vegetables and one pound of yam or brown rice or beans. Very quickly, my body began to clean out old, unwanted material—perhaps carcinogens, perhaps the leftover debris from chemo and radiation. The cleansing and detoxing happened in cycles, every few weeks in some other area of my body and with some new symptom—from pains, to phlegm, to loose stools.

After three years on a complete healing program that addressed her body, mind, and spirit, Dale went in for a CT scan—and her cancer was completely gone. That scan was in 1980, more than thirty years ago, and she has been cancer-free ever since. Since then, she has trained as a nutritionist and now helps other cancer patients develop comprehensive body-mind-spirit healing plans.

EAT ORGANIC FOODS TO DETOXIFY

The majority of Radical Remission survivors talk about the importance of ridding their bodies of all the chemicals and toxins we are exposed to in our world today. Scientists know that various things can cause a healthy cell to become cancerous, including bacteria, viruses, genetic mutations, and, of course, toxins. Researchers also know that certain toxins, such as nicotine, asbestos, and formaldehyde, definitively cause cancer; however, there are many other chemicals we are exposed to every day that scientists are still unsure about, such as pesticides and genetically modified organisms (GMOs). It took scientists over fifty years to prove that nicotine causes lung cancer, and it may take them that long, or longer, to determine whether or not pesticides and GMOs are making us sick.

In one alarming recent study, childhood cancers were associated with mothers who used common household or garden pesticides during the prenatal period.[23] A similar study showed that breast cancer patients had significantly higher levels of pesticides in their breast tissue compared to the breast tissue of women with benign breast tumors.[24] Unfortunately, it may take another fifty studies like these before scientists officially declare that certain pesticides cause cancer. In the meantime, most Radical Remission survivors choose to err on the side of caution by buying only organic fruits and vegetables. This appears to be a wise choice, since a recent study that looked at 240 different organic food studies concluded that organic food is 30 percent less likely to contain pesticides.[25]

IN ADDITION TO eating organic foods, a brief fast or cleanse can help speed up the detoxification of pesticides, heavy metals, and other toxins from the body. Fasting is one of the oldest medical treatments on record, and it has been documented in nearly every religious and traditional medicine system for the past three thousand years. It is considered by many health practitioners to be a natural way of clearing out infections and detoxifying the body, especially because—when done safely—it sets off a powerful domino effect of healthy changes in the body.

For example, studies have shown that brief fasts can help eliminate bacterial infections, reduce cholesterol, and slow the aging process.[26] A similar study showed that just twenty-four hours of fasting can kick off a major, internal detoxification process that cleans out entire organ systems and increases numbers of bacteria-fighting immune cells.[27] In terms of cancer, one pilot study showed that going on a short fast while having chemotherapy significantly increased the effectiveness of the chemo while also decreasing its side effects,[28] and some researchers hypothesize that eliminating all food sources of glucose through fasting may be an effective way to "starve" cancer cells.[29]

During my research trip around the world, I met many alternative health practitioners who use fasting as part of their recommended treatment for cancer patients. The director of one such fasting/cleansing program describes the health benefits this way:

Fasting is a wonderful vehicle for ridding the body of toxins that have accumulated and for improving the functioning of the waste disposal system in our bodies, so that we don't accumulate further toxins. . . . If I were diagnosed with cancer, I would go on a long-term fast, myself. . . . First, I'd want to get rid of the toxins, and then I'd want to [begin to] eat toxin-free [i.e., organic] food. . . . I'd want to fast [in order] to cleanse the tissues and to starve a fast-growing malignant tumor. It's the same thing that the chemotherapy and all the [conventional] therapies do. . . . Fasting is a natural way to go about it. . . . With most animals and organisms, when they're very ill, they stop eating. That's nature's way of doing this.

As this fasting director correctly points out, animals instinctively fast when they are sick. In fact, humans appear to be the only species that forces itself to eat instead. When animals start feeling sick, they typically stop eating and find a quiet, protected place to rest until they are well. During this time, they may sip water or eat a few bitter grasses (again, to help detoxify), but they will not resume eating until they feel better. For humans, our immediate loss of appetite when we feel ill indicates that we may also have this instinctual, self-healing mechanism asking us not to eat for a while in order to activate an internal detoxification process. Because some cancers have already been linked to bacteria and viruses (e.g., the human papillomavirus [HPV] has been linked to cervical cancer and *H. pylori* bacteria has been linked to stomach cancer), it may therefore make sense for cancer patients to go on a medically supervised, brief fast in order to help rid their bodies of any underlying viruses or bacteria that may be lingering.

When I was in Thailand for my research, I was intrigued enough to try a weeklong fast, which included a bit of watermelon and carrot juice, nightly vegetable broth, daily colonics, fiber shakes, herbs, and vitamins. I get incredibly cranky when I am hungry, so I figured I would make it about six hours before caving. However, I was happily surprised that the well-timed fiber shakes kept my hunger pangs at bay all week, while the juice, broth, and vitamins gave me the micronutrients my body needed. Without going into any of the gory details regarding something called "mucoid plaque" (you can google it), suffice it to say I finished the week in tremendous awe of my body's ability to detoxify itself via fasting—and as a newly converted vegetarian. I now try to do that fast once a year as a way of "spring cleaning" my internal organs.

If the idea of fasting in order to help detoxify your body seems daunting, you may wish to start with a one-day fast of fresh vegetable juices, supplemented with psyllium husk fiber (e.g., Metamucil) every four to six hours to keep your hunger pangs away. Fasting like this one day per month is an easy way to detoxify your body. Remember, always speak to your doctor first in case your fast needs to be medically supervised.

DRINK FILTERED WATER

The fourth and final change that almost all of my Radical Remission research subjects make is to switch from soda, juice, and milk to drinking approximately eight glasses of water per day, making sure the water is as clean as possible. Water is our barest necessity when it comes to health. It makes up about 70 percent of the human body, and without it, we will die in about four days. Many of the alternative healers I have interviewed consider water to be a "master healer," with the power to flush out toxins, viruses, and bacteria and provide the body's cells with much-needed hydration.

As such, these healers recommend drinking natural spring water, because of its higher mineral content, and avoiding tap water, since it often contains chlorine, fluoride, and heavy metals, all of which have been associated with cancer in certain studies.[30] While much more research is needed before we can know definitively whether or not these contaminants are linked to cancer, the Radical Remission survivors I study once again choose to err on the side of caution, either by drinking spring water from bisphenol-A (BPA) free, at-home watercoolers or by installing home filtration systems for their tap water (e.g., reverse osmosis, carbon filter). However, such filtering also removes all the healthy minerals from your water, so it is wise to take a trace mineral supplement if you filter your water. I personally use a home filtration system attached to my kitchen sink that removes chlorine, fluoride, heavy metals, and other contaminants from my tap water, and I use this filtered water for both drinking and cooking.

———————

SO FAR, WE have explored the four main dietary changes that Radical Remission survivors make in order to help their bodies heal:

- reduce or eliminate sugar, meat, dairy, and refined foods,
- increase vegetable and fruit intake,
- eat organic foods, and
- drink filtered water.

I would now like to share with you the healing stories of "Ginni" and John, which vividly illustrate how—when Ginni and John were faced with breast and prostate cancer, respectively— they used these four strategies to try to heal their cancer. Both Ginni and John live in rural (yet different) parts of the United States; therefore, they were not in places where they could necessarily turn to an integrative oncologist or a nutritionist for guidance. Instead, they were left to do their own research, which they both did by reading endless books, poring through their local libraries, and doing selective Internet research. As you read their stories, I encourage you to keep an open mind. Although their choices may not match your own, they nevertheless found solutions that worked for their particular bodies.

⎯⎰ **Ginni's Story** ⎰⎯

Ginni was sixty when she found the lump in her breast. At that time, in 2007, she had been working diligently at her longtime job and was enjoying a quieter phase of life with her loving husband. Quiet, that is, until she found out she had breast cancer. Neither a mammogram nor an MRI could adequately diagnose her lump, but a core biopsy finally confirmed that it was indeed breast cancer. Her doctor scheduled an immediate lumpectomy, which is a minor surgery to remove only the tumor and not the whole breast, but unfortunately he did not get "clear margins," meaning that he was not able to remove the entire tumor during the surgery. In addition, some of Ginni's lymph nodes tested positive, meaning she had stage 3 (out of 4) breast cancer. Her doctor wanted her to have a second surgery to get clear margins and also remove many of her lymph nodes. He told her that, after the second surgery, she would need intensive chemotherapy followed by radiation treatment. And then he gave the worst news of all: her prognosis. In her calm, no-nonsense tone, Ginni recalls that fateful moment:

The doctor said to me, "After you get this [second] surgery done and have the chemo and radiation, we can give you five more years to live." And I thought, I want to live more than five years! . . . So, when the doctor said that, I got mad. I didn't say anything to him, but I got mad and I knew right then I wasn't doing it. I wasn't going to do it, because I had already talked to [my friend Ron] and I already had information [about alternative treatment options]. So, I kind of went out with an attitude of This isn't going to beat me. I'm going to do this.

Therefore, with as much bravery as she could muster, Ginni calmly refused the second surgery, the chemotherapy, and the radiation, even though there was still cancer present in her breast and her lymph nodes. Most cancer patients would be too afraid to refuse the recommended treatment like Ginni did, but she was actually more afraid of the second surgery, because she had read that removing lymph nodes could lead to lymphedema, which is a permanent and painful swelling of the arms and legs. More important, her friend Ron had recently healed his prostate cancer by radically changing his diet (and postponing any conventional medical treatment), so Ginni had at least one example to follow. She began reading as much as she could on the subject and was a bit overwhelmed by the huge amount of information she found. In fact, she was so confused about what she should and should not be eating that she simply stopped eating for a while:

I lost fifty pounds in two months, because for a while I didn't dare eat anymore. They [the books] were saying that your eating habits—certain things you eat—are worse for it [cancer]. So, I was afraid I was feeding it. So, I quit eating for a while. And then slowly I started putting the right foods back in. But because your system isn't used to that, you kind of get sick. So, it's a big change to your body. But then once you get used to eating like that, then that food is what tastes good, and the other food doesn't taste that good anymore—the processed food.

Before discussing with Ginni what the "right" foods were in her opinion, I wanted to hear more about how and why she had stopped eating. At this point in my research, I had already met quite a number of radical survivors and alternative healers who had used fasting as a part of their cancer treatments. However, it appeared that Ginni had fasted accidentally. "Was that like a fast?" I asked.

She replied:

*Well, yeah. Almost. Because I was scared I was going to eat the
wrong thing. And then I slowly started eating lettuce, and then
I brought other things into it. I wasn't sure what I was supposed
to be eating, but then I talked with Ron some more and got some
ideas of how to do this, because it's totally foreign to you, you
know. . . . It was almost good to stop [eating] and then start over.
But yeah, I lost a lot of weight. But I've gained it back [three
years later].*

Losing a lot of weight during a fast is very common and usually healthy and safe, as long as you are not terribly underweight to
begin with, which Ginni was not.

As is typical when breaking a fast, Ginni first ate easy-to-digest
foods, such as lettuce. Then she started adding other foods and
drinks—what she considered to be the right ones—back into her
diet. She based her decisions on the many books she was reading,
such as Patrick Quillin's *Beating Cancer with Nutrition* and Chris-
tina Pirello's *Cooking the Whole Foods Way*. Remember, Ginni was
living in rural America, with no integrative nutritionists or doctors
nearby. Therefore, she had to do all the research herself.

*I started with not eating sugar, flour, or dairy products. It was
mostly vegetables, fruit, and no red meat whatsoever—a little
chicken here or there, or fish, but I didn't do a steady diet of that.
It was mostly green stuff. And juicing cabbage is very important,
so I did that.*

Ginni also bought a watercooler for her home and started drinking large quantities of bottled instead of tap water. Not only was
this better for her health based on what she had read about chlo-
rinated tap water, but it tasted better, since her local tap water was

very "hard," having a high mineral content. She also cut out all soda, milk, and alcohol and only drank juice if she juiced it herself.

In addition to these dietary changes, she bought all organic food, if possible, and only bought frozen foods when fresh ones were not available. The decision to eat organic foods was very purposeful, because Ginni had read that chemicals and pesticides might be the cause of her cancer in the first place. She also switched from eating white and wheat breads to eating sprouted-grain breads, and she began taking breast-support vitamin supplements from her local health food store.

Like all the other Radical Remission survivors I study, Ginni did not do just one thing to get better; rather, she utilized all nine key factors in her healing process. So, in addition to changing her diet radically, she released stress by walking thirty to forty minutes per day, which was a new habit for her. In her opinion, stress is detrimental to the immune system, which is why she was determined to release it from her body. She also grew incredibly close to her sister during this time and greatly benefited from the additional social support her sister provided. When I asked Ginni about whether she had any spiritual beliefs and/or practices during this time, she replied:

> *Well, you trust in God, and how God gave you this immune system to get rid of diseases. So, if you have your immune system up to where it's supposed to be, your immune system can do all kinds of things. But if your immune system is poor, then the diseases will take over. And I really believed that. . . . And we go to church every Sunday, and I kind of think that I believed more after I got the cancer. It's like I thought about it more.*

For a year, Ginni kept strictly to her new regimen of eating whole foods (mostly vegetables), drinking bottled water, taking vitamin supplements, and walking every day—until one day she could not feel the lump anymore. She immediately went to see her doctor and he could not feel it either. They decided not to do a mammogram, since that had not been able to detect the lump initially (only a core biopsy had), and he instead instructed Ginni to continue monitoring herself with monthly self-exams. It has been over five years since her initial diagnosis. Her health is great, her lump is gone, and she has found no new lumps since then.

Due to the underlying fear that her cancer might someday return, Ginni has diligently stuck to her new diet. It has not been that hard for her, however, because she now gets an upset stomach whenever she eats any of her "old" foods, such as white pasta or anything fried. Her taste buds have also permanently changed: now she actually craves fruits and vegetables, and refined foods no longer appeal to her. Overall, her life has settled into a new shade of normal, where vegetables now reign supreme and refined foods are relics of the past. When I thanked Ginni for sharing her amazing story with me, she replied:

> I'm glad to share it, because I think it's a remarkable thing, and I wish more people would try something different. But people are scared, because chemo and radiation are the only things they know. . . . They don't understand how something like [changing your diet] can work.

According to Ginni, the changes she made worked for her because she was giving her body the healthy, pesticide-free food and water it needed in order for her immune system to operate optimally and therefore remove her cancer cells.

MEANWHILE, A FEW states away, a man named John was dealing with a situation similar to Ginni's. The difference is that John first tried all the medical treatment his doctors recommended for his advanced prostate cancer. Unfortunately, despite all that treatment, his cancer recurred—which is when he started looking into other options.

ᴄ᷾ John's Story ᷾ᴄ

In 1999, at the age of fifty, John was stuck in an extremely stressful financial situation after going through a long and difficult divorce. To top all that off, his prostate-specific antigen (PSA) blood level was quite high, which was very worrisome to his doctor. A needle biopsy confirmed that John indeed had prostate cancer (with a Gleason score of 5 [3 + 2]), a finding that was understandably very scary to him. Therefore, when his doctor recommended that he have a radical prostatectomy, in which the entire prostate is surgically removed, John instantly agreed. "I was like, 'Cut it out now. I mean, like tomorrow!'" he recalls. "I was scared to death."

After the successful surgery, John's PSA thankfully dropped to almost undetectable levels and therefore no additional hormone or radiation therapy was necessary. Relieved, John went on to enjoy almost six years of being cancer-free, although he struggled daily with the negative side effects of the surgery, which greatly affected both his normal urinary and sexual functions. During those six years, his routine PSA tests came back very low year after year, which made sense given that his cancer had supposedly been limited to his prostate—at least according to what his doctors had told him—and his prostate was now gone. (Note: After a man's prostate is fully removed, he can still have very low levels of PSA in his blood, caused by leftover, benign prostate cells.) Everything seemed to be fine—except for the side effects, of course—until 2005, when John's PSA began to climb rapidly, indicating that cancerous prostate cells had traveled outside his prostate at some point before the surgery and were now active in his body.

Because John was dealing with recurrent prostate cancer, his doctor had him do both hormone therapy and radiation therapy, both of which gave him very unpleasant side effects. The treatments lowered his PSA to a safe range while he was on them, but a few months after completing both therapies, his PSA began to rise yet again above the safe range. His doctors told him that he would therefore have to go back on the hormone therapy and, if the cancer ever formed a metastatic tumor somewhere else in his body, he would also have to start chemotherapy. To John, this news felt like a slow death sentence. He dreaded going back on the hormone therapy and dealing with its harsh side effects, and the fact that his PSA rose as soon as he went off the treatment made him feel like he was never going to be free of this disease:

> I went to a bookstore because I remembered seeing a book there on how we died. I wanted to figure out how prostate cancer progressed and how you eventually died from it. Instead, I found Patrick Quillin's book on beating cancer with nutrition. So, I thought, Hey, I'll give this a try, you know? So, upon reading his book I learned that cancer cells are obligate glucose metabolizers—that's what he calls them—which means they're sugar feeders. So, I immediately eliminated sugar from my life. Period. Cold turkey. . . . It took about two weeks before I got over the cravings for any kind of sugar, and then I went and had another PSA test—and I noticed that it had started to drop.

Thus began John's personal science experiment to save his life. He postponed the recommended hormone therapy in order to give dietary change a try, and for the next six months he kept a careful diary of everything he ate, trying his best to follow the book's numerous recommendations, while also reading as many reputable articles as he could find. Like Ginni, John did not know an integrative doctor or oncology nutritionist with whom he could work, so it was up to him to come up with his own integrative plan, which he did after exhaustive research. He decided to get his PSA tested every three months, which is the standard amount of time to wait between PSA tests. What he found shocked him: his PSA appeared to go up and down depending on what he ate or drank during the previous three months. He explains why he thinks this happened:

> *Testosterone is what makes the cancer "go," and sugar is what feeds it. So, the theory I've developed is starve the cancer and let my immune system kill it. I've been practicing that, and what I've found—the hard way—is [that] some foods contribute to my PSA rise and some don't. I started eating edamame—soybeans— because that's supposedly good for cancer [according to the book he was following]. But I started doing that and the PSA shot right up, way up. So, I quit the soybeans and, boom, [the PSA] dropped off.*

In other words, John learned early on what researchers have only recently discovered, that there is no such thing as one type of prostate or breast cancer but rather various subtypes that respond differently to different treatments.[31] For some breast and prostate cancer subtypes, organic, non-GMO edamame may have an anticancerous effect, but for other subtypes, it may promote the cancer.[32] John noticed a similar drop in PSA when he strained the lignans out of flax oil and consumed only the clear part of the oil. Through a meticulous process of trial and error, confirmed by his regular PSA tests, he has since developed a very particular diet for himself to keep his PSA under control. His recommended best practice is if you don't make, cook, or steam the food yourself, don't eat it. The only sweeteners he uses are crushed blueberries and stevia (a natural sweetener made from leaves of the stevia plant). A book he read indicated that agave nectar would be a safe sweetener for cancer patients, but John saw that when he used it, it made his PSA rise, so he cut it out of his diet.

As the months went by, John converted his food diary and PSA results into a line graph:

> I've got a graph that you wouldn't believe. It's up, down, up, down, up, down. I've been doing this every three months for years. . . . I also cut down—way down—on red meat, which I've learned has a harmful effect on my PSA. So, I try to limit myself to sockeye salmon and organic chicken breasts, but small amounts. And I'll still have a steak now and then, but not every day. . . . The problem is that red meat and dairy products suppress the immune system, from what I've read. . . . And I confirm that every time I go off and have a red wine and red meat at a conference every year. When I come back, my PSA shoots up again.

John has also eliminated all dairy products and simple carbohydrates, such as pasta and bread, and discovered that apples, beets, cherries, and grapes are too sugary for his PSA. (Interestingly, though, bananas and freshly squeezed orange juice are okay for him.) In terms of liquids, he has cut out all sugary beverages, drinks only filtered (reverse-osmosis) or carbonated water, and has limited his alcohol consumption to red wine. Staying on such a strict diet is not easy for John, which is why he allows his taste buds to have their favorite meal of steak and red wine at least once a year.

Like all the other Radical Remission survivors you will read about in this book, John did not do just one thing (e.g., diet change) to try to heal his cancer. In addition, he changed other aspects of his life. For example, he increased his exercise regimen—which was already two to three times per week—to daily, and doing so led him to shed twelve pounds, which he has never gained back. Thanks to a combination of yoga, hiking, and walking, he now feels like he's in the best shape of his life. John also began taking an immune-boosting supplement called ImmunoPower and drinking herbal essiac tea, which his friend had read was good for fighting cancer. He also tried acupuncture, which he still enjoys from time to time. Finally, he also did his best to manage stress and stay positive. As he describes:

> *I think a positive mind is* very *important. You know, your attitude. I'm just determined not to let this control me. I'm gonna control* it—*the cancer, that is. It's kind of like a cold that won't go away. I know it's there but I'm not afraid of it anymore. . . . Now it's an irritation—it irritates me [laughs]. . . . And when I get stressed out, I can fall into my meditation or my breathing. I can breathe things away. . . . I can tune out.*

While the focus of my research is asking people why they think they healed, I also ask survivors if they have any thoughts about what might *cause* cancer, or about what might have caused their cancer in particular. When I asked John this question, he immediately replied:

> *I think everybody has cancer. And I think everybody's immune system fights it differently. If your nutrition is such that it lowers*

*your immune system, then you're going to get it. Your body's
constantly fighting off the cancer, but at some point it's gonna
overwhelm your immune system. And that depends on how strong
your immune system is. If you've got a weak immune system,
you don't have a chance. And everything you put in your mouth
affects the level of your immune system—plus the other factors,
you know, exercise and all of that. . . . And the problem with our
American diet is [that] everything's loaded with sugar, so you're
constantly feeding the cancer that everybody* has. *If your immune
system can't keep up with it, sooner or later it's gonna get ya.*

John went on to say that he believes he got his particular cancer
because he was eating tons of sugar at that time and was also
coming off a ten-year period of intense stress, all of which he feels
weakened his immune system. As a result, his immune system just
"couldn't keep up."

In retrospect, John says—had he known what he knows now—
he would have done things differently. To begin with, he would
have tried to diagnose his cancer using a combination of ultrasound, PSA, and other blood tests, as opposed to a needle biopsy. In
addition, he would never have agreed to the surgery, which removed
his prostate, because it has caused severe and permanent side effects
in both his urinary function (i.e., occasional incontinence) and
sexual function (i.e., inability to have an erection without drugs
or injections). He also would not have agreed to the radiation or
hormone therapy, both of which he feels were very harsh on his
immune system. Instead of those treatments, he would have tried
from the beginning to control his PSA through dietary changes,
immune-boosting supplements, regular exercise, and consciously
taking steps to reduce stress in his life. As John sees it:

It's really simple. Sugar feeds [cancer]. Testosterone makes it go.
And your immune system controls it—or kills it. So, you've got to
boost your immune system and lower your sugar. It's that simple.

As he told me this, I noticed a bit of resignation in John's tone, so I asked him whether he enjoyed the new diet he was on. He immediately responded:

I hate it! I don't like not being able to eat whatever I want.
I don't like not being able to party with friends like I would
like to. It's just a constant, daily regimen that I hate. In fact, I
wear a couple of skull rings to remind me that, if you don't have
discipline, it will kill you. . . . I have a nice lady friend that
loves to travel, and I enjoy traveling with her. So, I want to stick
around awhile. . . . You've got to have something to live for.

It has been more than thirteen years since John's initial diagnosis of prostate cancer and more than seven years since his recurrence and the start of his new diet. He still sends me occasional e-mails updating me on his latest PSA level, and I always have to smile when I think of him hating his strict diet yet loving life more.

Action Steps

I hope John's and Ginni's stories of healing have convinced you that, if you want to help heal your body, you need to pay attention to what you put into your body. I know that making dietary changes can be emotionally stressful, whether due to a need to gain satisfaction from food or due to body image and weight loss issues. Some people will read this chapter and immediately sign up for a seven-day fast or cleanse, throw out all sugary and refined foods from their pantries, and fill their fridges with organic fruits and vegetables. If that is you, kudos.

However, if you are more like me, you may need to take smaller, even baby steps toward the anticancer diet described in this chapter. Over the past ten years, I have gradually moved toward these four dietary changes, allowing me not to feel deprived of foods that satisfy me while also giving me the time to learn how to cook healthier options. If baby steps are what you need, here are some to get you started:

- *Reduce slowly.* Start with one less sweet, one less portion of meat, one less serving of dairy, and one less refined food per day. Start exploring healthier alternatives to these foods, such as coconut ice cream, pinto beans, hemp milk, and quinoa.

- *Eat at least one vegetable or fruit with every meal,* and build up from there until half of every meal is veggies and fruits.

- *Prioritize what organic foods to buy*—certainly meat and dairy, but also those fruits and vegetables that absorb the most pesticides: apples, celery, tomatoes, mushrooms, etc. Over time, your grocery bill should stay the same as you replace expensive meat with organic fruits and veggies.

- *Start your morning with a glass of filtered water with lemon juice* to help detoxify your body. First, buy a simple pitcher filter, and then save up for a home filtration system.

After you complete these steps, you can move on to bigger changes, such as investing in a juicer and juicing organic vegetables, first once a week and eventually once a day. Then consider putting yourself on a two-week elimination diet, where you temporarily eliminate all non-fruit sugar, meat, eggs, dairy, gluten, soy, alcohol, and caffeine. After the two weeks, add each food back into your diet one by one, spacing them out every three days. By doing this, you may find that certain foods make you feel terrible when you add them back in, while others give you no issues. Finally, if and when you feel ready, you can look into doing a one-, three-, or seven-day cleanse and/or fast, which may need to be medically supervised depending on your particular health status.

———

WHILE THERE IS no guarantee that changing your diet like Ginni and John did will reverse your cancer completely, after a decade of researching thousands of Radical Remission cases, I am thoroughly convinced that Hippocrates was absolutely right: food is medicine. Eating more organic vegetables and fruits while reducing sugar, meat, dairy, and refined food products can only help your body to heal—and, in fact, it may turn out to be the only medicine you need. Hippocrates believed that healthy food and water should be the first medicine given, and surgery and drugs should only be used as absolute last resorts. Two thousand years later, we have somehow managed to turn that order on its head: we first look to medications and surgery to heal our sick bodies, instead of the powerful medicine we already take three times a day: our food.

CHAPTER 2

TAKING CONTROL OF YOUR HEALTH

Action is the foundational key to all success.
—PABLO PICASSO

The word "patient" comes from the Latin word *pati,* which means both "to suffer" and "to allow" or "to submit." In today's world, medical patients are not necessarily expected to suffer, but they are expected to allow or submit. Having worked as a counselor at various hospitals and oncologists' offices, I know firsthand that the patients who listen and follow instructions are considered "good" patients, while the "annoying" patients are those who ask a lot of questions, bring in their own research, or—worst of all—challenge their doctors' orders. Such patients are labeled annoying because most of the world still operates from the Newtonian mind-set of medicine, where doctors are seen as the only "mechanics" who know how to fix the "machine" of the body when it breaks down.

Radical Remission survivors approach healing from a different perspective, where taking control of your healing is not only considered good but is actually essential for the healing process. From what I have learned, taking control of your health involves three things: taking an active (versus passive) role in your health, being willing to make changes in your life, and being able to deal with resistance. After we explore these three concepts in depth, we will experience the healing story of a Radical Remission survivor who took control of his health at the eleventh hour, followed by some simple steps you can start taking right now in order to gain more control over your health.

NOT BEING PASSIVE

While modern medicine may view the body as a machine whose parts can sometimes break, alternative healers view things a bit differently. They see the body as a sophisticated organism that intertwines the physical body with the nonphysical mind and soul. In addition, they view the body as something that can function quite well as long as you take proper care of it, the mind, and the spirit. It is kind of like taking care of your car. You can either drive it around recklessly, scratching it and denting it and never taking it in for an oil change, or you can drive it gently, providing it with high-quality fuel and oil, and cleaning it regularly. When you look at it this way, the most influential player in this scenario is neither the car nor the car's mechanic, but the *driver*.

In the world of Western medicine, we have been trained to be such "good" patients that we have forgotten we are actually the ones driving our "cars" (bodies). We have only rudimentary knowledge about how to care for our bodies, and when they do break down—often due to nothing more than lack of care—we hand over all responsibility for fixing the problem to our doctors, instead of thinking about how we could change the way we care for our bodies. In return, our doctors typically give us pills that either mask our symptoms without resolving the underlying problem or resolve the problem yet create side effects.

Radical Remission survivors are the "annoying" patients who

do not automatically do whatever their doctors tell them to do. To extend the metaphor, they are car fanatics who research the best fuel and motor oil, clean and wax their cars regularly, and never miss an oil change. When it comes to their health, they take a very active role in their healing process.

One such Radical Remission survivor, who quickly learned to be active instead of passive with regard to her healing, is Sun Hee Lee, a Korean-born mother of two. When Sun Hee was diagnosed with stage 4 ovarian cancer, she had a large ovarian tumor as well as a "malignant pleural effusion," meaning she had cancerous fluid in her chest cavity. As a result of the pressure from this fluid, the middle lobe of her right lung had partially collapsed, and her lower lobe was close to a total collapse. Most patients with this diagnosis and these symptoms live only about six months. As the native English-speaker in the family, Sun Hee's husband, Sarto Schickel, describes how they immediately took an active role in her healing:

> *My wife is now more than five years past her original diagnosis and is living a normal life. This is an extremely rare and unexpected result for someone with stage 4 ovarian cancer. She achieved this by using both conventional treatments—surgery and limited chemotherapy—and alternative therapies, including Gerson therapy and a macrobiotic diet. If we hadn't decided to take her healing into our own hands by blending conventional and alternative therapies, I believe she wouldn't be here today. We both strongly believe that if doctors and patients would embrace conventional treatments and alternative dietary and detoxification approaches together, in a new integrative healing paradigm, then more radical recoveries could perhaps be accomplished.*

While Sun Hee's doctors were surprised that she took such an active role in her healing, many of the alternative healers I study expect such behavior from their patients, and some even require it. In their opinion, people cannot fully heal unless they get in touch with their own inner power. One such healer is a kahuna healer from Hawaii named Serge Kahili King, who believes that, while healers can be of assistance, healing must ultimately come from inside the patient:

> *All power comes from within. The body heals itself. No one [i.e., a healer] can take control of another person's autonomic system. It can't be done. [Healers] can, however, help a person subconsciously to find their own source and strength—so it's more like assistance. The body has the power [to heal], but there's so much tension in the way that it can't apply that power. So, subconsciously, it's possible for [healers] to give suggestions that will help the subconscious or the body-mind to relax and stimulate its own healing powers. [Healers] might even be able to use energy to help amplify the body's normal healing powers. But the healing comes from within. . . . It doesn't require an esoteric master at all.*

In other words, Serge believes that cancer patients can choose to use outside doctors or healers as helpers in the healing process, but true and deep healing always comes as a result of the patient taking an active role in the process.

WILLINGNESS TO CHANGE

The second aspect of taking control of one's healing is the idea that, in order for healing to occur, you must be willing to analyze your life and make changes, even if those changes are time consuming or emotionally difficult. This is different from the modern medicine paradigm, which rarely takes the time to analyze the unique lifestyle of each patient and, instead, tends to prescribe quick-fix pills or sometimes surgery to address a problem.

One longtime breast cancer survivor, who quickly realized she needed to make changes in her life in order to regain her health, is Elyn Jacobs. Elyn was diagnosed with stage 1 breast cancer at the age of forty-five, when her children were just three and four years old. As soon as she was out of surgery, she was already researching additional things she could do to help her body heal. She had watched her mother go through endless chemotherapy only to die of breast cancer a few years afterward, and Elyn was determined not to let the same thing happen to her:

> *My immune system never seemed to be quite right—colds were frequent and persistent. There were other red flags as well. Once diagnosed, I realized that I had to make some changes, to take control of my health. I read everything I could get my hands on. I tweaked my diet, worked on my stress, and embraced the use of supplements to boost my immune system. Seven years later, I have no detectable cancer cells and my immune system, while not perfect, seems to be very much up and running.*

One of the hardest changes Elyn had to make during her healing journey was, for the sake of her health, not returning to her stressful job as a bond trader. Although making this change was difficult at first, she now enjoys quality time at home with her husband and two boys, and she also coaches cancer patients on how to integrate alternative and complementary approaches into their conventional treatments.

The healers I study also believe that patients must be willing to go inward and carefully examine the ways they can change in order to regain their health. One of these healers is Bryan McMahon, an

American-born practitioner of Traditional Chinese Medicine who studied, lives, and practices in Shanghai, China. Bryan believes cancer patients must ultimately make internal changes in order to fully balance their chi, or life-force energy:

> *I believe that Radical Remission, or the sudden improvement of any type of illness, is not necessarily something that a doctor can give a patient. It's something that a patient must give themselves. . . . The inclusion of some type of insight practice into your own state is absolutely essential for people who are facing any type of illness. Because it's only through this tangible feeling and understanding of what is the* actual *state that you are in—energetically and physically—that people can actually begin to say "Wow, I really have ignored my life for so long. I really have been trying to do too much. I really have been too controlling." It's only through that type of practice that people can begin to do the internal maintenance that's required to really bring about permanent change in the dynamics of their chi mechanisms. Instead of [the chi] going completely out and up, we start to see the energy return, start to come back in to where it needs to be.*

From the perspective of Bryan and other alternative healers, examining your habits and lifestyle, and then making appropriate changes, invites more chi—also known as prana—into the body. Bringing more chi into the body is considered a very good thing to do because a constant and unrestricted flow of chi is believed not only to keep us healthy but also to keep us alive (i.e., in Traditional Chinese Medicine, when you have no more chi left in your body, the body dies). Therefore, being willing to make changes that increase your inflow of chi is seen as a key factor in the healing process.

Johnnie's Co-Workers over the Years

Maintenance

Elijah (Ed) Strater
Paul Hurt
Toney Earl Williamson
Gregory Fritz
Reginald Royster
David Jordan
Ferber Herndon
Johnny Wilkerson
Al Foye

Ervin Green
David Bumpass
Danny Holloway
Harry Chavis
Roger Wilkerson
George Cozart
Andre McCaden
Rodney Hunt

Administration

Bruce Smith
Deborah Bass
Brenda Thornton
Lorraine Satterwhite
Charmaine Cypress
Barbara Sneed
Tonya Burwell

Fran Terry
Patricia Bass
Katrina Watts
Michelle Campbell
Michelle Moss
Xavier L. Wortham
ReJean Tate

Board Members

Willie S. Darby
William Cozart
Robert Wainwright
Elizabeth Watts
S. I. Roberson
Brian E. Hicks
L. H. Perry

Dr. Abram Liles
Patricia Kiesow
Delores Lyons
Dr. John W. Watson Sr.
Charlie F. Jones
John W. Beach

DEALING WITH RESISTANCE

The third aspect of taking control of one's health is the notion that taking control often means dealing with criticism from others, and therefore the person needs to have a strong enough backbone to be able to deal with that resistance. As mentioned earlier, patients who take control of their healing are typically labeled as "annoying" patients by the conventional medical system, and as a result, they are not always treated well by members of their medical team.

One Radical Remission survivor who had to face this kind of resistance is "Janice." Janice was diagnosed with stage 4 cervical cancer in 1985, and she first had a full hysterectomy followed by radiation therapy. Although less than a year later the radiation treatment was not helping, Janice refused to believe she was going to die and instead began researching complementary medicine techniques she could start trying:

> *When I was in the hospital, the doctors and nurses spent two hours a day for two months trying to convince me that I was going to die, that there was no hope, that I had to accept this. I told them I did not accept it. I understood what they were saying. I understood their statistics. I understood the prognosis. However, I was determined to stay focused on the possibility that my health was assured, that I would be cured. . . . And I do believe my level of control positively affected my healing. . . . The doctors and nurses said these [complementary treatments] wouldn't have any effect. They thought our efforts were ridiculous and that we should just accept my fate and get prepared to die. If I hadn't had the strong intuitive feeling that I would live, and perhaps if I weren't a bit of a rebel by temperament, I would have listened to them and wouldn't be here now to tell my story.*

After the radiation failed to help Janice's cancer, her doctors sent her home on hospice care. This meant she was finally free from the daily resistance she had faced in the hospital, and she could now focus all her energy on increasing her complementary treatments, including diet changes, colonics, and the use of essential oils as supplements. She was completely cancer-free just a few years later and has been healthy ever since—almost thirty years later.

Sometimes, the resistance you encounter when you begin taking control of your own healing is internal as opposed to external. This internal resistance usually takes the form of self-doubt or fear, and it is yet another hurdle most radical survivors have to face at one point or another. One such survivor is Vanessa Lukes from New Zealand, who was a cancer patient before becoming a qigong healer. Qigong is a gentle meditation and movement practice that has been shown to have many health benefits, and tai chi is one of its most famous subtypes. Vanessa describes what it was like when she was diagnosed with advanced colon cancer at the young age of thirty:

I started reading, first about the physical, the body, nutrition. And I just crossed things off, [because] I'd always been what I thought was healthy—super fit, active, and eating healthy foods. So, I thought, Well, there's got to be more to it than this. . . . It's often the hardest way, but you've got to go inside. You can't go out, because there's actually nobody out there who can do it [i.e., heal] for you. And that's actually quite scary, because you're the only person who can do it, but you've got to go inward and keep going in. . . . It's quite tricky for people to know what to do, but I feel that everyone will work out their own path and see things clearly for what they are. If it doesn't work, try something else.

Although Vanessa had to overcome some internal fear and doubt about finding her own route to healing, her perseverance eventually

led her to the inward practice of qigong, which she ended up studying for many years under the tutelage of Master Yuan Tze. Today,
she is happily cancer-free and offers qigong classes to cancer patients
all over New Zealand.

RESEARCH ON TAKING CONTROL

In this chapter so far, we have seen how Radical Remission survivors and alternative healers value the trait of taking control of the
healing process. The question I would like to turn to now is "Does
science also value that trait?"

In terms of the research behind taking control of your health,
I would be remiss if I did not mention the famous type C study.
You have probably heard about the type A personality, someone
who is high-strung, competitive, and has a tendency toward anger.
This compares to the type B, someone who is more laid-back and
relaxed. These terms stem from studies done in the 1950s, and they
inspired another study in the 1980s that looked at a third type of
personality—type C—which the researchers described as someone
who is overly passive, does not stand up for him- or herself, and
always tries to please others (basically, the opposite of a type A).
This single study found a strong association between a type C personality and developing cancer, and it showed that having a type
C personality may weaken your immune system.[1] As you might
imagine, this study created a wave of controversy, and since then
numerous other studies have both reconfirmed the type C–cancer
connection and refuted it—so, the jury is still out. However, the
most recent studies all seem to indicate that feeling helpless—
much more so than being passive or pleasing—is what weakens
your immune system, and it also decreases survival time in cancer
patients.[2]

If feeling helpless appears to reduce your chances of surviving cancer, what might the opposite—*taking control* of your cancer treatment—do for you? In observational studies that looked at people who have overcome cancer against all odds, "taking control of one's health" is almost always a common thread. I certainly found this to be true in my own research, which is why I have dedicated an entire chapter to the topic. A similar study found that Radical Remission survivors "assumed responsibility for all aspects of their lives, including recovery; thus, medical personnel were often used as consultants."[3] Another study found they all "bucked the system" when it came to taking control of their health,[4] while yet another found they experienced both an "increase in personal autonomy and a decrease in helplessness" before they healed.[5] In other words, whenever researchers take a closer look at Radical Remission survivors, they discovered the survivors all took control over their health and became very active in the decision-making process.

In addition to these observational studies, prospective studies have shown that taking control of your health may lead to longer survival times for cancer patients. A "prospective" study follows people over a period of months or years, while an "observational" study looks at people at one particular point in time. In one such prospective study, which studied the effects of group psychotherapy on cancer survival, researchers followed a number of stage 4 cancer patients over a period of one year. Interestingly, they found that those cancer patients who were willing and able to take action to improve their psychological well-being (by regularly attending therapy sessions, doing the assigned homework, and making the recommended changes) were the ones who lived the longest.[6]

Another prospective study looked at stage 4 cancer patients who turned into Radical Remission survivors and compared them to stage 4 patients who did not survive. Among other things, this study found that the survivor group had high levels of autonomy—the ability to control what happened in their own lives—while the non-survivors had low levels of autonomy.[7] Finally, another study compared a group of Radical Remission survivors to a group who had also survived cancer but in a way that was statistically expected. Interestingly, the researchers found that the Radical Remission survivors were *more* passive than the expected survivors at the time of diagnosis but much *less* passive than them at the time of remission.[8] In other words, the people who made the biggest shift away from being passive and toward taking an active role in their health were the ones who were most likely to turn into Radical Remission survivors.

So, from the studies that show that being helpless can weaken our immune systems to the observational and prospective studies that show that taking control is a commonality among Radical Remission cancer survivors, it seems safe to conclude that taking an active as opposed to passive role in your health is an important—if not crucial—step in the body's self-healing process.

———

SHIN TERAYAMA IS a Radical Remission survivor who greatly values the trait of taking control of one's healing, although he did not start taking control of his healing process until *after* he was sent home on hospice care. His odds-defying recovery from advanced kidney cancer is a beautiful example of how it is never too late to take control of your health.

—૭ Shin's Story ૭—

As a teenager growing up in 1950s, postwar Japan, Shin Terayama was expected to work hard in school, stay out of trouble, and respect his elders. During this time, he also met one of his first loves: the cello. Shin had a natural talent for music, and he happily practiced his cello every day until he graduated from college, when his heavy workload made it impossible for him to keep up with his cello playing. He began working twelve to fifteen hours a day, a lifestyle that continued well into his working life.

Over the next few decades, Shin's career flourished with a series of job promotions; he also married an adoring woman and together they had three beloved children. However, his work demands increased each year, and by the time he was in his forties, he was working around the clock as the president of his own consulting firm:

> When I was forty-six, my regular time was from five to eight in the morning [giving] a presentation as the president of the company. Nine A.M. to twelve P.M. [was spent] visiting some companies. And in the afternoon, I had some conversations with the management of the company. In the evening, from six to nine P.M., I talked to the staff. And I returned to my office at nine P.M., and I worked until two A.M. to prepare for the next day. Every day!

While it may sound extreme, Shin's work schedule was not unusual for Japanese men at that time; this was how successful Japanese businessmen were expected to spend their lives. Therefore, Shin remembers feeling happy at that time, at least in the sense that he was proud of his career and his family. However, while he may have felt okay about his schedule, his body did not. At age forty-six, he started feeling deeply fatigued, even though his doctor could not find anything wrong in his test results.

Over the next year and a half Shin saw numerous doctors at various top-notch hospitals, but all of his blood tests kept coming back normal. Nevertheless, his health was slowly deteriorating, with his fatigue worsening and blood beginning to appear in his urine once a month. One day he had an appointment with a new doctor who specialized in internal medicine. Because Shin's was the final appointment of the day, this doctor was able to take some extra time to examine him. For the first time in a year and a half, a doctor actually touched Shin's body instead of just looking at test results on a sheet of paper. The doctor palpated Shin's stomach, chest, and back for any potential problems, which is how he discovered that Shin's right kidney was enlarged and sore to the touch. The doctor immediately sent him to a urologist, who—after performing an ultrasound—found that Shin had a very large tumor on his right kidney.

Shin's doctors urged him to have surgery immediately to remove the tumor, especially because there was a chance it could be cancerous. However, Shin said he was under way too much pressure at work to take an entire month off. So, he postponed the surgery for several months while he kept at his grueling work schedule. After five months of postponing like this, his health was so bad he was running a constant fever and could barely walk. At this point, his wife and doctor absolutely insisted he have surgery—and Shin finally agreed.

During the surgery, the doctors discovered that Shin's tumor had become so big they now needed to remove his entire right kidney, which they did. They also learned from the pathology report that he had advanced renal cell cancer (a.k.a. kidney cancer). However, in Japan at that time, it was a common practice not to tell cancer patients they had cancer, especially if they had a serious prognosis like Shin did. Therefore, when Shin awoke and asked his doctor whether or not the tumor was cancerous, his doctor evasively replied, "It's somewhere in the middle." In reality, Shin's doctor and

wife knew the truth: Shin had less than a year to live if the chemotherapy and radiation treatments were not effective.

After Shin had recovered from the surgery, his doctor told him
that he would need some special "injections" to make sure the
tumor cells did not spread to other parts of his body. Still oblivious,
Shin took these injections without question, not knowing they were
actually cisplatin, a very strong form of chemotherapy:

> *The chemotherapy started two weeks after my operation—*
> *well, the injections [started]. And I [got them] two weeks*
> *continuously, from Monday to Friday and Monday to Friday.*
> *And my hair all fell out, as usual, but still I didn't know that it*
> *was chemotherapy. And several times I asked my doctor, "It's too*
> *strong. What's the name of this injection?" And he said, "You're*
> *so nervous. Don't worry about that. It's a good one."*

When the strong "injections" were finished, Shin's doctor told
him he still needed more treatment, this time a special "high-energy
beta-ray" treatment. In reality, this was just the standard radiation
treatment given to cancer patients. So, Shin stayed on in the hospital and received a total of thirty radiation treatments, taking breaks
whenever the side effects became too severe. After the chemotherapy and radiation, a whole-body scan revealed that Shin's cancer
had spread to his right lung and rectum, and his doctor warned his
wife that he had only a few months to live.

Between the inpatient chemotherapy and inpatient radiation,
Shin had now spent about five months in the hospital. During this
time, more than five hundred friends and colleagues visited him, os-
tensibly to say hello and cheer him up, yet in reality they were there
to say their good-byes—because, at this point, everyone knew the
truth except Shin. Then, one night Shin had a dream:

At the beginning of March, I had a very strange dream that I was lying in a coffin. And I was looking from above—it was a funeral! And when the lid of the coffin closed, I returned to my body and shouted, "I'm still alive!" It was completely a dream, but something changed [afterward]. My sense of smell increased very strongly.

Shin awoke from that powerful dream not only wanting to fight for his life, but also with a superhuman sense of smell that made staying in the hospital close to unbearable. The hospital had strong disinfectant odors, plus Shin was staying in a large room with six other patients, separated only by sliding curtains—and the various odors in the room were excruciating for his new sense of smell. One night, not long after his coffin dream, the smell in his room was so severe that he snuck out in the middle of the night to go to the roof for some fresh air. Having brought his blanket with him, he lay down on the roof and breathed in the clean air for hours, letting it fill his lungs and nose. When a group of harried nurses finally burst out onto the roof, they began shouting at him not to jump. As much as Shin tried to explain that he was not trying to commit suicide, the nurses did not believe him. Later that morning, his doctor was very displeased with him:

The nurses had reported to my doctor that I was trying to jump off from the rooftop to [commit] suicide. I didn't want that—only to avoid the smell. . . . My doctor came by early in the morning and he was very angry, very upset about my behavior. . . . He said if I wanted to return to my home, it was my choice. He wanted to avoid his responsibility to the patient, because my name was a little bit famous at that time. If I did [commit suicide], the newspapers would write about it.

Although Shin did not realize it at the time, sneaking off to the roof ended up being the moment that saved his life, because it allowed him to leave the hospital and begin his own healing process. At this point, his wife decided to tell him the truth, that he had very advanced kidney cancer. Shin was not that surprised, because he had been guessing for the last few months that he probably had cancer. Now, faced with the harsh truth, he decided he would rather die at home with his wife and children than in a pungent hospital room. So, his doctors released him to hospice care and stopped all his cancer treatment. They fully expected Shin to die in one to three months, especially given the fact that he still had cancer in his rectum and right lung.

When he finally arrived home, Shin was in such bad shape that he was only able to walk with the help of a walker and had to be fed intravenously. Thankfully, though, he was still able to drink:

> After I returned to my home, I couldn't drink tap water. It smelled. So, I tried to make good water from tap water, to change it. And I had a charcoal carbon [filter], and I used it in a bucket one night. It was very good, changing the water! . . . So, then I noticed [that] water is very important, and I asked my son to buy mineral water. . . . I knew about the wonderful [benefits] of fasting, and I had no fear about it. So, I drank water and it was a fasting, actually, because I couldn't eat anything at that time—only water every day. Even [though] I was not treated by any medical treatment, my body was gradually getting better and better. That's the first step—only water.

When Shin says he was fasting, he means his digestive system was not breaking down any food, because his intravenous (IV) nutrition was sending all the nutrients directly into his bloodstream.

Therefore, all his digestive organs—his liver, pancreas, stomach, gallbladder, and large and small intestines—were effectively resting during this time. He was essentially on a water fast. As mentioned in chapter 1, the vast majority of mammals will go on a water fast whenever they are sick, and studies have shown that doing so for a few days allows your digestive organs to clean out any viruses, bacteria, or dead cells.[9] The organs can do this because they are not busy digesting three meals a day. Therefore, in Shin's case, being on IV nutrition was a blessing in disguise because it allowed him to go on a water fast.

The morning after returning home from the hospital, Shin awoke before sunrise and was overwhelmed with gratitude about being alive to see another day. By this point, he had realized the gravity of his illness and fully believed he might die at any time:

> *When I woke up in the morning and saw it getting light outside, I said, "I'm still alive! Today is a new day!" . . . I was living in a second floor apartment with my wife and three children, and I wanted to see the sunrise. The rooftop is [on the] eighth floor and so I went to the rooftop by using the elevator. And when I saw the sunlight, it was so wonderful. Then I tried to see it [the] next day and [the] next day. And every day I said to the sun, "I'm still alive!" And when I saw the sun, I [realized] that the only energy we receive from the universe is the sun. . . . It was the first time I had noticed [this] kind of a thing.*

During our interview, Shin's voice was filled with wonder as he described going to see the sunrise day after day. By accepting the fact that he was going to die soon, each new morning was truly a gift for him. All fear of dying had left his mind and body, and it was replaced by immense gratitude for any additional breaths he

was given. As he sat up there on the roof of his apartment building each morning, soaking up the warm energy of the sunlight, he
began to notice something subtle about his breathing:

> *I noticed that my body was getting better by exhaling. Exhaling*
> *and automatically inhaling. . . . And then one day I tried to put*
> *a tone with it, like this [sings a single note while exhaling]. . . .*
> *Before my disease, [a yoga teacher] said to me, "Your chakras are*
> *closed, and your aura is very dirty." . . . So I tried using tones,*
> *and when I touched [certain] points on my body, the tone got*
> *louder. So that was the point of the chakra! And I found seven*
> *main chakras by doing [this] kind of exhaling every morning,*
> *just experimenting. . . . Seven chakras are, for a musician [sings*
> *the seven notes of a major scale]. And so I tried to connect each*
> *chakra from bottom to [top].*

In other words, Shin was combining one of his talents—music—
with two of his new healing modalities: exhaling and watching the
sunrise. As he experimented with singing a single note during an
exhale, he discovered that certain notes reverberated more strongly
in certain areas of his body. For example, a lower note resonated
more strongly in the center of his chest, while a slightly higher
note resonated more strongly in the center of his throat. Without
knowing it, he was discovering the seven energy centers of the body,
or chakras, as they are called in yoga. (Shin has since studied the
chakra system in depth.) These energy centers start at the base of
the spine and move up to the top of the head, and they are thought
to be very important in the flow of energy throughout the entire
body. Also, if one or more of your chakras are closed or partially
blocked, the theory is that illness or dysfunction will result. By
exhaling and singing vibrating tones while watching the sunrise,

Shin was helping to clear out and energize his seven chakras, even though he did not realize it at the time.

One day when Shin awoke before the sunrise, he noticed that the birds were already singing, which piqued his curiosity:

I [wondered,] "Why are the birds singing? When do the birds begin to sing?" That was my question. And so I got up ten minutes [earlier], twenty minutes [earlier]—still they were singing. Thirty minutes—still singing. And then I got up one hour before sunrise, and it was completely quiet. . . . I tried to see when they started singing and it was forty-two minutes before the sunrise. Every day! . . . So, after I checked when the birds [were] beginning to sing, I had nothing to do until the sunrise. So, I did [this] kind of exhaling for forty minutes.

Shin timed the birds for a month, and he noticed that, without fail, they started chirping forty-two minutes before the sun rose, even though the time of the sunrise changed slightly each day. A scientist by training, Shin was not content to accept that birds simply begin singing forty-two minutes before the sun rises; he wanted to know *why*. He had an idea about it that he wanted to investigate, so he asked his son to buy a cylinder of oxygen from the local pharmacy. Shin's family happened to own three pet birds, whose cage they covered at night to help the birds sleep. One night Shin decided to stay up late to conduct his experiment. Around midnight, he silently released some oxygen into the birds' room. A few minutes later, the birds began chirping. After a few more minutes, presumably when the oxygen had dissipated, the birds grew silent again and slept. Excited by this development, Shin waited until around 2:30 A.M. and then silently released more oxygen. As predicted, the birds began singing again and stopped a few minutes afterward. Finally, later that morning, the birds began singing yet again, this time forty-two minutes before the sunrise, and they chirped continuously until the sun rose.

Shin's theory was that the birds started singing forty-two minutes before the sun rises because they were responding to the oxygen the trees started to emit in the morning. During photosynthesis, which can only happen in the presence of light, trees absorb carbon dioxide from the air and release oxygen. Trees do not photosynthesize at night, but they do start emitting oxygen as soon as it starts to get light out in the morning—which is approximately forty-two minutes before the sun rises. Scientists are still not sure why birds sing more in the morning as opposed to other times of the day,[10] but Shin's best guess is that singing allows birds to breathe in lots of fresh oxygen from the trees, which are just beginning their day's worth of photosynthesis. Shin's miniature science experiment convinced him that the air is especially healthy to breathe during the forty-two minutes leading up to sunrise, and this was even more important to him since he had cancer metastases in his right lung.

In addition to giving fresh air to the cancer in his lung every morning, Shin started giving it something else: love. This decision came about after he realized he had seriously mistreated his body during his working life:

> When I returned to my home, I tried to find the reason why
> I [was] suffering from cancer, and I [realized] I created this
> cancer myself. I created it because I worked so hard, and I didn't
> sleep. I created it! So, I thought that cancer was my child. And I
> sent love to my cancer, and pain decreased and I could sleep fine.
> [The] next morning when I got up, my mind, my head, [my]
> brain was so clear that I didn't use any painkillers. . . . So, I

stopped [using] painkillers and instead of that, when I had pain,
I [said], "Oh, thank you very much for saying you are hurting.
I love you, my child." I touched this [points to his kidney] and
said to my cancer, "I love you, I love you, I love you." And pain
decreased! That's why I sent love to my cancer always, from
morning till night. . . . Unconditional love, that's unconditional
love. I said [to it], "Thank you very much for existing."

Shin's decision to send unconditional love to his cancer, which he viewed as his "sick child," is highly unusual. Most cancer patients think about "killing" their cancer cells, which they see as hostile invaders that need to be destroyed. Quite to the contrary, Shin saw his cancer as something to which he himself had contributed, because of how he had neglected his body (and mind and spirit) during his stressful working years. Therefore, just as one would care for a sick, neglected child, he viewed his cancer in a loving, almost apologetic way, mentally sending love to it multiple times a day. I explained to Shin that many of the cancer patients I work with would be afraid to send love to their cancer, out of fear that it might cause it to grow faster. Shin believes the opposite actually happens—that when given love, cancer cells "heal" and revert to the healthy cells they once were:

Conventional medicine comes from hunting tribes, like Anglo-
Saxons. . . . In the history of medicine, doctors found out about
bacteria and viruses, and they tried to kill them. They tried
to find some kind of medicine to kill them, like a weapon. . . .
[Western doctors] try to kill cancer. I once met [the man who
discovered] the natural killer cell. So, I said to him, "You
say 'natural killer cell,' but I think 'natural healing cell.'"
Conventional medicine [tries] to kill, always kill, kill, kill. I didn't

kill my cancer. I loved it. The most important thing I learned is
that cancer is my body. It's not an enemy; it's still my body.

So, this is how Shin lived his life for a few months: feeling grateful for each new morning, drinking clean mineral water, waking up every morning to breathe and sing with the birds before sunrise, and sending love to his cancer each day. After about two months of this daily ritual, something unexpected happened as he was watching the sunrise. An amazing feeling of energy began emanating from the base of his spine and then slowly moved upward along his spine toward his head. In the world of yoga, this is known as a "kundalini awakening" experience, in which a coiled ball of energy that supposedly has lain dormant at the base of the spine is one day awoken and released. Shin had never heard of any of these terms before, but after this unforgettable experience, he read up on them:

Two months after [doing the breathing in the mornings], I had
[an] experience with kundalini. No one told me [this] kind
of thing could happen. I couldn't stop it. . . . When I had the
experience of kundalini arising from [my] spine, after that I
could see auras very easily. . . . I felt nothingness in my body,
emptiness . . . especially [in my] brain. . . . And after I had the
experience with kundalini, the [amount of light frequency] I
could see was widened. . . . I can see much more in the dark now.
No need for light!

In yoga theory, an aura is a colorful field of light that surrounds every person as a result of our electromagnetic nature (e.g., the human heart is electrical and sends out an electrical impulse with each beat). This aura, or energy field, is something that cannot be seen with the naked eye, just as one cannot visibly see the waves of energy in a microwave. However, some people have developed the ability to see these auras with their eyes, usually as a result of an intense meditation or yoga practice. Although Shin did not think of his morning sunrise ritual as a meditation practice, that is exactly what it was. His mind was quiet, he was focusing on his breath, and he was chanting tones in order to clear his chakras. Therefore, it is not surprising that after two months of doing this he experienced an awakening of kundalini energy in his spine, leaving him with a heightened visual ability.

After watching the sunrise each morning, Shin enjoyed quality time with his wife and three children, who at that time were ten, fourteen, and seventeen years old. Shin's health continued to improve little by little, and soon he began walking and eating normal food again. He greatly enjoyed not having to work eighteen-hour days; he had not experienced this lifestyle since he was a young boy. He worried that, if he continued to get better, he would eventually have to return to his grueling work schedule. Therefore, after a long talk with his wife, they decided she would continue with her work (because she truly enjoyed her career as a professor), and they would significantly cut down on their expenses, so Shin could stay completely focused on his healing. This gave him an incredible sense of relief, and it allowed him to expand upon his healing activities. One of those was returning to playing his beloved cello:

> *I had stopped my cello practice twenty-five years [earlier], and then . . . one of my teacher's [other students] asked me to come to his home and enjoy cello playing. I went there four months after I [was] discharged from the hospital. When I listened to the cello—Oh! It sounded very nice and it changed my emotions so much—especially [my] chakras open[ed] very easily by [the]*

cello's tone. And so, I decided to practice cello again every day. So,
cello was my medicine—without any side effects! [laughs]

Another thing Shin did for his health was to visit an alternative
healing center in the Japanese mountains. He went there for one
week each month, not only to breathe in the fresh mountain air and
eat their organic food, but also to take a soak in their natural, hot
mineral springs. As a former volcano chain, Japan has hot springs
like this all across the country, and it is culturally believed that
soaking in them is very beneficial to your health. Overall, research
studies suggest that soaking in hot mineral springs can have either
a neutral or positive effect on one's health and may be especially
beneficial to those with arthritis, chronic pain, or dermatologi-
cal conditions.[11] Two theories about why the springs may produce
such positive results are that, first, the water is rich with important
minerals, such as iron and calcium, and second, the hot water helps
to raise your core body temperature slightly, thereby mimicking a
fever and helping your body "burn off" bacteria and viruses. Shin
describes his time spent at the alternative healing center this way:

[When I was sick] a most effective thing was to go to a hot spring.
It's to warm up and detoxify the body. It's very wonderful. . . .
Our bodies [are] always making toxins, because we are moving.
With movement, we are making toxins. . . . The most important
thing [for detoxifying] is the surface of skin, to open the pores
of the skin. And not just by sweating. . . . Also by relaxing we
can open the pores. This is very, very important. . . . And by
breathing [exhales deeply], we can relax.

After his relaxing trips to this mountainside health center, Shin
would return home and continue with his healing activities. One of

these was giving himself a home enema as often as once a week. He also tried to eat healthfully, sticking to mostly whole grains, fresh fish, and lots of fruits and vegetables. However, he purposefully chose not to "go crazy" with his food. For example, one very rigid diet that many cancer patients undertake is called the macrobiotic diet, which actually originated in Japan. One of the things this diet eliminates is coffee, which made Shin pause:

You know about macrobiotic food? So, I tried to use it. And [the] macrobiotic [diet] knows something truth[ful] about food. But most people in Western countries, including Japan, are trying to do microbiotic, not macrobiotic. [laughs] They stick to a small thing—not to eat something, not to eat salt, or not to drink coffee. I like coffee. Because I know coffee is [a] wonderful thing to activate [the] brain. . . . If people feel the truth of the food, that's most important.

In other words, Shin tries to stick to an overall healthy diet that makes his body feel good, as opposed to becoming obsessed with which specific foods to eat or not eat. He also purposefully does not take any vitamin supplements or herbs, as his intuition tells him he should try to get all his nutrients from whole foods. In addition, while he eats those whole foods, he focuses on chewing the food slowly while feeling grateful for the food he has been given.

As time went on, Shin's doctors—who were very surprised that he had not yet died—decided to monitor him carefully. However, their preference was to do monthly CT scans, which Shin intuitively felt were unhealthy due to their radiation. Instead, Shin agreed to do quarterly blood tests and CT scans every six months. As the months went by, his blood tests and CT scans showed gradual and steady improvement, much to his doctors' surprise. Nevertheless, three years after he was sent home on hospice care, the scans showed that he still had some cancer in his body.

At this time, Shin's story of miraculous survival had spread, and he was being asked to speak and write about his healing techniques. Even though he still had cancer in his body, people found it incredible that he was given three months to live and yet was still alive three years later. One of the organizations that asked him to come speak was the Findhorn Foundation spiritual community in Scotland. This is an educational center dedicated to spiritual and consciousness teaching, and the directors invited Shin to spend a month learning and sharing at their retreat center. Shin's wife did not want him to go away for that long, but Shin's intuition told him he should go. So, he packed a bag and his cello and went off to spend a month in a country he had never visited, to be with people he had never met. As soon as he arrived, he was embraced into the small community, and they treated him like a long-lost uncle. He was incredibly moved by this wonderful surge of love from perfect strangers, and he especially appreciated all the hugs he received— something that is not very common in Japanese culture:

> When I went to Findhorn, people hugged me so much! Whenever they saw me, every time [they said], "Hello, Shin!" Morning hug, afternoon hug, evening hug, and also goodnight hug! Unbelievable. Strong, unconditional love, from morning till night. . . . In our Japanese culture, we only say [things]; we don't hug. But hugging is very important. Hugging communication uses the auric layer. . . . So, we can communicate using energy exchange by using this auric layer.

Shin elaborated on his theory that hugging is a powerful way to transfer energy to another person, because the two people's auras

merge for that brief moment of a hug. Many of the alternative healers I interview would agree with this theory. While Shin had sent as
much love as he could to his own cancer during the past three years,
he had not necessarily received a lot of loving energy from outside
sources, because Japan is so conservative when it comes to physical
affection. Therefore, all the hugging and unconditional love he received from strangers in Scotland was a new but welcome source of
energy and support for Shin.

When he returned to Tokyo after his month at Findhorn, it was
coincidentally time for his biyearly CT scan. Much to his surprise,
his cancer was no longer visible on the scan. While the cancer could
have been slowly receding over the previous six months since his last
scan, Shin credits his month at Findhorn with being the final step
his body needed to remove his cancer completely. When I asked
him what he thinks happened during that month to cause this final
healing, he replied without hesitation: "Love."

Shin has been full of love—and free of cancer—since 1988, and
it has been more than twenty-five years since he was sent home on
hospice care. Instead of dying, Shin took control of his healing one
step at a time, and today he dedicates his time to helping other
cancer patients learn how they can heal their bodies, minds, and
spirits. In his free time, he plays the cello and laughs with his many
grandchildren.

Action Steps

Shin Terayama is a great example of someone who took control
of his healing, although it was perhaps easier for him to do this
because his doctors had already run out of suggestions by the time
he was sent home on hospice care. Many cancer patients are not in
Shin's position. Instead, they are often bombarded with conflicting
advice from every person they meet, which makes it confusing and

difficult to begin taking control of their healing. Their oncologists may be telling them to eat ice cream and steak in order to gain weight before chemo, while their nutritionists may be telling them to give up dairy and meat in order to create a noninflammatory internal state. Their acupuncturists may recommend plant-based herbs, while their doctors may be saying no to all supplements. Their therapists may be asking them to delve into their past, while their energy healers may be asking them to release it.

If you or someone you love is in this kind of situation, there really is only one solution: become the lead decision maker. Ask your various "helpers"—your doctors, therapists, nutritionists, etc.—to explain the rationale behind their recommendations. Do not be afraid to ask as many questions as you want. Request books or articles you can read on the subject in order to become better informed, keeping in mind that nothing in this world is ever black and white. Although you may never catch up on the amount of knowledge and training your doctor, nutritionist, or acupuncturist has in his or her area of expertise, you should at least be able to understand what that person is doing to your body, so you can be fully on board with whatever treatment you—not they—choose.

In addition, here are some simple things you can do to make sure you are taking control of your health, whether you are trying to prevent cancer or heal from it:

- Find a general practitioner who does not get annoyed when you ask questions or bring in your own research. Ideally, you want one who will respect you for taking such an active role in your healing. Once you have found that doctor, expand your search to include any other health practitioner you need, such as acupuncturists, naturopaths, psychologists, nutritionists, energy healers, and massage therapists.

- Learn how to research. Staying informed is one of the most powerful things you can do for your health, so make it a goal to read at least one health-related article per week from a source you enjoy and trust. In addition, begin to familiarize yourself with the U.S. National Library of Medicine's search engine, called PubMed, which can be found at Pubmed.gov. This is an online database of almost every peer-reviewed medical article, and you will want to learn how to read and understand at least the abstracts of these articles so you can discuss them with your doctor, should the need arise.

- Take out a sheet of paper and write down these three headings: physical, mental/emotional, and spiritual. Then spend ten or more minutes carefully analyzing and writing down any aspect of these three areas of your life that could use some improvement. Be reflective and honest with yourself. Then circle the items that would bring about the biggest improvement in your health and happiness, and tackle those first.

- Find an accountability partner. You will undoubtedly run into some external or internal criticism as you begin to take control of your health by making changes. To better withstand this criticism, ask someone who will *not* be critical to hold you accountable for the changes you are hoping to make, and offer to do the same for him or her in return.

I HOPE THESE suggestions give you some ideas about how to start taking control of your health, if that is something you wish to do. While Shin's healing story shows us that it is never too late to get involved in the healing process, I sincerely hope you won't wait until you are on hospice care to start taking an active role in your health. More important, I hope you are never a "patient" again— neither one who suffers nor one who passively submits—but instead you always decide to take an active and engaged role in your life, health, and happiness.

CHAPTER 3

FOLLOWING YOUR INTUITION

In vital matters, the decision should come from the unconscious, from somewhere within ourselves.

—SIGMUND FREUD

In many ways, humans have lost touch with their instincts. We used to be hunters and gatherers—people who could sense when a storm was coming or feel when a grizzly bear was nearby. Our sense of smell also used to be much more highly developed, as it expertly guided us toward safe food and away from poisons. When we got sick, we listened to our bodies by allowing a fever to burn off the illness and by not eating for a few days. Today, things are quite different. We rely on whatever The Weather Channel tells us, we eat whatever processed foods we find in the supermarket, and we take whatever medicine our doctors give us.

There are two potential problems with relying on such outside sources of information, though. First, the sources could be wrong. For example, commercials in the 1950s showed doctors in white coats promoting the health benefits of cigarettes, while margarine—with all its trans fat—was touted as a "healthier" alternative to butter. These examples show us that others do not always know what is best for us. Second, instincts are a lot like multiplication tables: if you don't use them, you lose them. Along this line, researchers believe that our sense of smell has diminished over the past few centuries because we no longer need it to survive, as safe food is now so abundant in our grocery stores and restaurants.[1] However, by not keeping our sense of smell well honed, we have lost the ability to detect *new* toxins in our environment, such as cancer-causing chemicals in our food, air, and water.

And then there is intuition, that famous sixth sense or instinct that seems to come from a deeper place. Many people would argue that we have lost this as well. For example, there are records of our ancestors following the intuitive guidance they received from dreams, and thousand-year-old yogic texts describing meditation exercises that can help increase our intuitive abilities. Although I was not expecting it, "following your intuition" has ended up being one of the nine most common factors of Radical Remission among the people I research. I remember, on my fiftieth or so interview of these survivors, thinking, *There it is again!* However, now that I have done further research on intuition, I am no longer surprised but thrilled to have been reintroduced to this "lost" sense of ours, which has the ability to help steer us away from danger and onto the path of recovery.

In this chapter, we will first explore three aspects of intuition as described by the Radical Remission survivors I study, followed by the story of a woman whose intuition played a key role in the healing of her pancreatic cancer. Finally, you will find a list of simple action steps that you can start taking right now to help you rediscover your innate, sixth sense of intuition.

THE BODY KNOWS WHAT IT NEEDS TO HEAL

The Radical Remission survivors I study believe the body has an innate, intuitive knowledge about what it needs in order to heal, and it can often also let you know why it got sick in the first place. It is because of this that many Radical Remission survivors believe it is vital to check in with your intuition before making any sort of healing plan. Interestingly, this belief goes against typical Western medicine thinking, which usually removes patients from the planning process while the expert doctors determine what is wrong with their bodies and how to fix it.

One of the alternative healers I studied, who firmly believes the body intuitively knows what it needs in order to heal, is "Maya" Karen Sorensen, a BodyTalk practitioner from Hawaii. BodyTalk is a form of energy medicine that uses the principles of energy kinesiology and muscle monitoring to figure out where the root problems are located in the body, what's causing them, and how they can be released quickly. In this way, Maya works directly with the intuition of her patients' bodies. She describes her healing in this way:

BodyTalk is speed healing, because the body wants to be whole and knows how to be whole. But sometimes it needs to be reconnected to its innate knowledge. The body can heal very instantly; it's our belief system that makes us think that it takes a long time to heal. Using energy medicine kind of bypasses the belief system, because it taps into the client's deeper, innate wisdom of the body.

Similarly, another healer I researched believes the body naturally knows how to return to wellness. Derek O'Neill is a Radical Remission cancer survivor himself who later became a healer and now encourages the cancer patients with whom he works to access their intuition:

If the mind is allowed to quiet down, it will know what it needs to do in order to get well again. It's a built-in system that every being has. . . . So, cancer is actually only a messenger. It's not a be-all and end-all, in my opinion. It's a messenger to say that something has gone negative, something is out of alignment. Find out what that something is, and you will note that the energetics of your own body will begin to correct that system.

Once cancer patients become aware of the ways in which their lives have become out of balance, Derek encourages them to make addressing those imbalances an integral part of their healing plan.

THE MANY WAYS TO ACCESS INTUITION

The second aspect of following intuition is that there is no one "right" way to access your intuition. For some people, their intuition comes to them through an internal voice of deep knowing; for others, it comes more as a physical feeling in their bodies, such as a warning pang in their guts; for still others, their intuition speaks to them in their dreams, their meditations, their journals, or through serendipitous "coincidences," such as bumping into a friend who told them exactly the information they needed to hear at exactly the right time. All these methods are valid ways to access your intuition, and the more often you access it, the clearer the messages will be.

One Radical Remission survivor who used dreams to access her intuition for healing was Wanda Easter Burch. When Wanda was forty-two, she began having vivid dreams warning her that she had breast cancer, even though her mammogram was clear and an ultrasound was inconclusive. Nevertheless, she insisted on having a needle biopsy, and that is when her dreams proved to be true: she indeed had aggressive breast cancer.

After her diagnosis, Wanda began to study dream interpretation more deeply, and she blended meditation, drawing, and poetry into her conventional treatments of surgery and chemotherapy. She describes her use of intuitive dream work this way:

> *Before and after my radical surgery and aggressive chemotherapy, my dreams presented images that provided personal, creative material. Dreaming—and selective mining of dream imagery—empowers the mind, spirit, and body. Dream work encourages dialogue with the inner physician—a constantly streaming, two-way message center that speaks to us, knows us best, and offers gateways to healing beyond the hospital or doctor's office. There are no artificial boundaries in a dream, nor a limit on the varieties of creative and healing artistic expression that can emerge.[2]*

Wanda used dreams to help her figure out which foods to eat during chemotherapy, which emotional patterns to release, and which conventional medicine treatments to consider. She has now been cancer-free for over twenty-three years.

Another Radical Remission survivor who used dreams to access her intuition was Nancy. On May 1, 2006, Nancy was just about to turn sixty-five when biopsy results came back showing that she had breast cancer. Her tumor was too big for a lumpectomy, so her doctor recommended a full mastectomy followed by radiation therapy and the estrogen-reducing pill tamoxifen. However, Nancy's intuition told her to try alternative methods first, so she politely turned down the surgery and all other conventional treatments. Listening to her intuition, especially her dreams, turned out to be a pivotal part of her healing:

> *On May 5 [four days after her diagnosis] I had two dreams. . . . In the second dream, my son-in-law was looking for Spray 'n*

Wash to treat a dark red stain on our old, well-worn tablecloth. I told him where it was, but he couldn't find it. After much searching, I found it right on the table and went ahead and sprayed the stains, which began to dissolve. In real life, [he] is a skilled orthopedic surgeon. I believe my intuition was telling me that I could heal this cancer without surgery, but it would take time and effort, and I'd find the solution right there in my own, well-worn, much-used, much-loved body.[3]

After putting together a healing plan that encompassed dietary, exercise, herbal, emotional, spiritual, and energetic treatments, Nancy was declared cancer-free by her doctor just sixteen months later. She remains cancer-free to this day and is certainly glad she listened to her intuition.

EVERYONE HAS A DIFFERENT CHANGE THEY NEED TO MAKE

The third aspect of following intuition is the idea that every person may have a different change they need to make in order to heal his or her cancer, and that is why checking in with your intuition can be so vital to your recovery. For example, I met one cancer survivor whose intuition told her she had to quit the job she hated in order to get well. Another person's intuition told him he had to move to a different climate in order to heal, and yet another person's intuition told her she needed to start exercising again. The alternative healers whose work I study agree with this idea of trusting your own unique intuition. They tell me repeatedly that every person has a different change they must make in order to restore balance to their systems. For some people, that may mean changing their diets, but for others, it may mean changing their marriages.

This idea goes against current Western medicine thinking, which aims to find a single cause for a disease and a single cure for it. In the case of bacterial infections, this goal is realistic: we can try to determine the single bacterium that has infected the body and then try to develop a single antibiotic that will destroy that bacterium. However, with a more complex disease such as cancer, which has already been shown to have multiple causes (toxins, viruses, bacteria, genetic mutation, mitochondria damage, etc.), finding a single cure may not be so realistic. In this case, then, it would make sense that some cancer patients would benefit greatly from making a particular change (e.g., radical diet change) while other cancer patients would not.

That's when intuition can be extremely helpful: when you are trying to figure out the particular change *your* body-mind-spirit needs in order to heal. Gemma Bond is a Radical Remission survivor who was diagnosed with ovarian cancer in 2011. After agreeing to a hysterectomy, during which her uterus and ovaries were surgically removed, her intuition strongly told her to refuse the recommended chemotherapy. Instead, she began exploring alternative therapies, such as intravenous vitamin C and ozone therapy. She also read as many books as she could find about alternative cancer treatment:

In one of the many books I have read, the author—a cancer survivor himself—suggests that anybody with cancer sit quietly with their cancer and then ask why it has come, and then ask it what needs to be done in order for it to leave. So, I did that. I sat quietly with my cancer and I thought, Why have you come? *I had led such a healthy physical life—I'd exercised, I'd eaten organic, I'd fed my four children what I thought was great, healthy food . . . but the answer really screamed back at me,* You have no joy in your life! You always have this really big to-do list, but where is your joy?

I had looked after my physical health, but I had really neglected my emotional health. And so, that has become the thing that I have worked on most in my healing, my emotional health rather than my physical health—although I have tweaked that as well.

Thanks to this intuitive insight, Gemma began addressing her emotional health by adding more joy to her life and deepening her connection with spirit. Only six months after her diagnosis, her tumor markers were back down to within a normal range, and she is still cancer-free to this day.

An energy healer based in London's Hale Clinic named Danira Caleta purposefully begins teaching cancer patients how to access their intuition in her very first healing session with them, so they can understand the specific ways in which their health has gone out of balance:

I teach [my patients] to actually turn on that switch in the unconscious, which is faith. In quantum healing, they call it "the doctor within." It's like a light switch. And I teach them how to do this. . . . Your body's on your side. It does actually give you a warning. It does tell us, "Look, there's something not quite right here." But most people don't listen and they put it off, thinking, Oh, it'll just go away. *So, one has to listen to one's body. . . . Cancer is about a journey to teach us many things about ourselves. It really forces us to examine how we're living.*

In Danira's opinion, when you use your intuition to listen to your body to figure out the particular change you need to make, healing will follow naturally.

THE RESEARCH ON INTUITION

While unfortunately there has not been a lot of research conducted on intuition specifically, researchers have made important discoveries that relate indirectly to intuition. The first discovery was that humans appear to have two very different "operating systems."[4] System one is the quick, instinctual, and often subconscious way of operating; it is controlled by the right side of the brain and by other parts of the brain that have been around since prehistoric times, known as the "limbic" and "reptilian" parts. System two is the slower, more analytical, and conscious way of operating; it is controlled by the left side of the brain and by newer parts of the brain that have only developed since prehistoric times, also known as the "neocortex." Researchers have found that intuition is part of system one, which is why it comes on so rapidly and often does not make rational sense to us. In other words, intuitive decisions are not things we think through carefully, with reason, but rather choices that arise quickly, out of instinct.

Second, scientists have discovered that over a hundred million neurons—the type of cells found in your brain—also exist inside the human digestive tract, which explains why people often say they have a "gut feeling" about something. This is because the gut, with all its millions of neurons, can actually think and feel just like the brain can.[5] Even more interesting has been the discovery that this "second brain" in your gut can act *independently* of the brain, meaning that your gut can decide to stop digesting food and send you a sudden, intuitive pang of warning without any input from your brain. So far, the gut is the only organ that has been discovered to have this independent operating ability.

All of this leads us to the fact that we now have a scientific explanation for why people so often decide to go with their gut when making a decision. People also feel pangs of anxiety or stress in their guts, but this is also related to intuition, because it is the body's way of saying, "Stop what you're doing. This situation is not healthy for you." So, your gut can communicate that it wants you to remove yourself from a stressful or anxious situation, just as it can communicate to you that *that one* is the house you should buy.

But why, exactly, should we trust a gut instinct? One reason is because researchers have found that system one often knows the right answer long before system two does. For example, in one study, researchers asked their subjects to play a card game where the goal was to win the most money. What the study subjects did not realize, however, is that the game was rigged from the start. There were two stacks of cards to choose from; one was rigged to provide big wins followed by big losses, while the other deck was set up to provide small gains but almost no losses. It took about fifty cards before the subjects said they had a hunch about which deck was safer and about eighty cards before they could actually explain the difference between the two decks. What is most fascinating is that after only *ten* cards, the sweat glands on the subjects' palms opened slightly every time they reached for a card in the dangerous deck. It was also around the tenth card that the subjects started to favor the safer deck, without being consciously aware they were doing so.[6] In other words, long before the analytical brain could explain what was going on, the subjects' bodily intuition knew where there was danger and guided them toward safety.

A similar study looked at people's ability to predict whether a picture was behind curtain number one or curtain number two (though this was done on a computer, so there were no actual curtains involved). Just like with the card study, the researchers measured the subjects' subtle physiological responses. Remarkably, they found that the subjects' bodies were able to predict the correct curtain two to three seconds *before* the computer had even decided which curtain to use.[7] The subjects did not always follow through with what their slightly sweaty palms were telling them to do, but the slightly sweaty palms were almost always right; in fact, they even had the ability to predict the future (by those two to three seconds). For gamblers who would like to have the ability to predict a certain card, this study suggests they should work on heightening their sense of intuition to such a degree that they can recognize when the sweat glands on their palms have opened up.

Finally, there is another set of studies that gives us yet another reason we should trust our intuition. These studies have found that, when it comes to making major life decisions, such as which house to buy or which person to marry, trusting your intuition leads to better outcomes than trusting your logical, thinking brain. In one such study, car buyers who had plenty of time to pore over all the information about their various car choices were later found to be satisfied with their purchase only 25 percent of the time. Meanwhile, those buyers who made a quick, intuitive decision about their car purchases were found to be satisfied with their purchases 60 percent of the time.[8] In three similar experiments, subjects were either given time to think about a complex problem or distracted and then asked to make a quick decision. Across the board, the subjects who were asked to make quick, intuitive decisions were the ones who made the best decisions overall.[9] In other words, these studies indicate that it is best to trust your intuition when it comes to making complex life decisions, while it is better to use your slower, more analytical brain for solving simpler problems.

While I was surprised to have intuition come up over and over again during my research of Radical Remission cancer survivors, these studies tell me that I should not be surprised at all, because our intuition often knows what's best for us even when our thinking minds do not yet understand what's going on. That's because intuition operates from the part of our brains that developed at a time when hidden dangers could jump out at us at any moment, such as a tiger hiding behind bushes. This part of the brain became highly skilled at sensing immediate danger as well as places of safety. However, because most of us now (thankfully) live a relatively safe day-to-day existence, that part of our brains is not triggered very often, and when it is, we are not familiar with it, so we tend to ignore its messages. However, we all still have it, and the Radical Remission survivors I study have learned how to harness its power.

IN TODAY'S WORLD, talking about following your intuition can make people think you are "woo-woo." That is certainly what happened with Susan Koehler. Susan's intuition came roaring up inside her when she was diagnosed with stage 4 pancreatic cancer, and everyone thought she was crazy for listening to it. As you read her complete healing story, I invite you to think about times in your life when your intuition has suddenly kicked in. Have you ever felt a pang in your stomach that made you pick up the phone and call someone just at the right time? Did the next major step in your life ever come to you in a flash of inspired creativity or through a beautiful dream? As you will see in Susan's story, we shouldn't ignore these flashes of intuition, because they often have important—perhaps even life-saving—information to tell us.

—⚬ Susan's Story ⚬—

When Susan Koehler was fifty-four, she started coughing every once in a while, even though she did not have a cold or flu. It started very slowly at first and then increased in frequency until, a few months later, it had become bothersome enough that she went to see her doctor:

Prior to what happened to me, I very much believed in Western medicine or allopathic medicine. If something was wrong, I always went to a doctor to have anything treated. So, about March of 2007 I went to the doctor because I had a cough that didn't seem to be getting better. And they started giving me all kinds of cough suppressants. Maybe six weeks later I went back to the doctor and I had some discomfort on my right side, just below my ribcage. The cough hadn't gotten better, despite the antibiotic that they'd given me.

Because the antibiotic and cough suppressants were not working, Susan's doctor ordered a chest x-ray, followed by a CAT scan, and then decided that she wanted a lung specialist to interpret the scan results. By the time Susan was sent to the lung specialist, her cough had been going on for almost a year, which was more of an annoyance to her than anything. Before sending her to the specialist, though, her primary doctor prepared her by saying that she might have one of three things going on with her lungs. It could either be histoplasmosis (a fungal infection) or sarcoidosis—with its collection of benign nodules—or, in the worst-case scenario, her doctor subtly implied that it could be lung cancer, but this was incredibly unlikely given that Susan had never been a smoker or been exposed to airborne chemicals (at least that she knew of). Her doctor expected it to be the first option, a fungal infection.

So, with a little bit of trepidation, Susan went to see the lung specialist in August of 2007. After another round of testing, the specialist—along with two other radiologists whom the specialist had asked to double-check her scans—came in to give her the heavy news. According to their expert eyes, they believed the nodules in her lungs were actually metastases (distant tumors) of a primary cancer located elsewhere in her body. Before this news could properly sink in, they had already begun more testing to try to find the location of her primary cancer. She had a colonoscopy—it was clear. She had an endoscopy—also clear. She had an abdominal ultrasound—clear as well. Finally, Susan's gynecologist persuaded her to request a whole body PET scan, which would instantly "light up" any cancerous hot spots. The other doctors agreed that this was the next best step, and so she drank the radioactive glucose and lay still for the thirty-minute PET scan.

When her doctors came in to give her the results, their faces were long and serious. Of all the organs in her body that could have "lit up" with cancer, it was unfortunately her pancreas that had lit up, along with her lungs. They told her she had late-stage pancreatic cancer with metastases to the lungs and, even with all their recommended treatment, she probably had only a year or two to live. With her heart beating loudly in her head, Susan tried to focus as they started explaining that she needed immediate surgery, radiation, and chemotherapy. However, at this very moment, something entirely unexpected happened to her:

> *At that diagnosis, I was sitting on the [examination] table and I—are you ready for this one? I heard a little voice in my head! [laughs] I had never heard voices before. But I heard a voice that said,* Not that way, not this time. *[My doctor] told me that the diagnosis was very serious and that I needed to follow his exact rules and guidelines in order to get myself better. If not, I did not have a good prognosis. I smiled then, because a yoga teacher had once told me that if you smile, you can sense danger fifty feet away. The smile incensed the doctor, at which point he became*

more verbose and authoritarian. That's when I knew that the danger was there—in that diagnosis, in that office. I never told him that I was not going to do what he recommended. I simply slipped from the table and left the office.

Susan's doctors strongly objected to her decision not to follow their medical advice, and they warned her she was "making a big mistake" by not listening to their recommendations. Nevertheless, as soon as she heard that inner voice, she decided to let her intuition guide her completely. So, when she got home, she immediately called her boss and told her she needed to cut down to working only Tuesdays and Thursdays in her educational management position. Instinctively, she knew she would need at least three days a week to dedicate to her new "job," which was figuring out how to heal herself. Strangely enough, though, even during those first few days after the diagnosis, Susan was not that afraid:

When I got the diagnosis, I felt very strongly that I wasn't finished with my work. . . . That's why I needed to figure out how to get healthy, because I wasn't finished with the work I had to do in this lifetime.

With this strong will to live as her foundation, the next thing Susan's intuition told her to do was to dig out one of her old journals from years earlier. Her father, also a nonsmoker, had died of lung cancer seven years ago, and his father before him (who *had* been a smoker) had also died of lung cancer. When Susan's father was diagnosed, she began to wonder about the sources of disease, and in her exploration, she came across a book called *Why People Don't Heal and How They Can* by Caroline Myss, Ph.D. The book resonated with Susan, so she later studied with the author directly, taking many of her workshops and attending many of her lectures.

At the very first workshop Susan attended, Caroline Myss had invited a Native American shaman named Lench Archuleta to lead the opening exercise, and Susan was struck by his teachings on healing. That is why in 2004, after Susan's dad had died, she decided to attend one of Lench's seven-day spiritual retreats in Arizona. As she had done her whole life, she kept a daily journal of her experience while at the retreat, and this was the journal she now dug out of her files:

> In my journal that I kept while I was there [at Lench's retreat], I had written that Lench told me that I was "leaking energy from my chest" and that he knew that my father had died from lung cancer and that I was also going to take on the burden of that "dis-ease" so that I could heal the next seven generations. Because in the Native American tradition, if you heal something, you heal seven generations before you and seven generations in front of you. I wrote it down, but I really didn't take it seriously at all. Even when I started getting the cough, it still didn't register with me. But something clicked when they gave me the diagnosis of lung metastases.

Reading her old journal entry made Susan feel like perhaps there was something larger at play here, something that could heal not only herself but perhaps her whole family as well. So, the next thing she did was reach out to a local holistic doctor who was known for working with cancer patients. However, that doctor said Susan would have to go through an exhaustive series of tests and follow her treatment plan exactly, with absolutely no exceptions or additions. Susan's intuition once again told her this was not the right path for her, so she politely declined. After that, she did not go to anyone else for help; instead, she simply went to the library and began researching on her own, using her intuition as her one and only guide:

> *I tried to study everything that I could, anything that anybody had done that was alternative, including looking at diet or cleansing or those kinds of things. . . . Once I gathered all the information I thought I needed, the first thing that I did was work on getting my pH in balance, because my internal environment was highly acidic. . . . I was using pH strips to test my urine, and eventually I was testing urine and saliva so that I could bring myself into a more alkaline balance. . . . I was pulling things out [of my diet] and putting things back in until I could get myself stable.*

Like so many of the survivors featured in this book, Susan began her healing process by changing something physical—in this case, her diet. An alkalizing diet focuses on eating alkalizing (as opposed to acidic) meals in order to reduce overall inflammation in the body. In general, all fruits and vegetables eaten either raw or lightly steamed will have an alkalizing effect on the body, while meats, proteins, carbohydrates, sugars, dairy foods, and anything fried will have an acidic effect on the body. In her research, Susan tried to go back to the original source of the alkalizing diet, which led her to Edgar Cayce's writings on the subject. And while Susan had always considered herself a healthy eater, studying the alkalizing diet led her to cut almost all sugar from her diet:

> *When I started trying to cleanse and change things, I literally lost about twenty pounds. And I will admit that I looked kind of gray, and my family was concerned that I wasn't doing the right*

thing. But my husband was very supportive and just kept saying, "As long as you think you're doing what's right, then that's okay with me." And I think it was just a matter of my body bringing itself back into balance. I lost the weight and I just continued to do what I was doing, and then slowly the weight came back on. Now I weigh about the same as what I've always weighed.

In other words, even though Susan went through a period of feeling and looking worse after changing her diet in this way, her intuition told her she was doing the right thing for her body and she should stick with it. Eventually, the detoxification phase ended, and all the nutrients she was ingesting with her new, vegetable-rich diet started to be absorbed fully, allowing her weight to come back on and her color to return to her face. During this time, her intuition also told her *not* to take vitamin or herbal supplements, because she felt her body would be better served if it received those nutrients directly from food.

Susan next turned her attention to exercise, because she intuitively felt that the breathing aspect of exercise would be important for her lung metastases:

I started walking every single day—not because of the exercise, because I've always been an exerciser, but [because] I felt that I really needed to connect with earth energy and be breathing in fresh air and not be working out in a gym or somewhere else. So, I started walking every day, first thirty minutes and then I worked up probably to about an hour-long walk every morning, even in the wintertime—and I live in upstate New York.

Between her new diet and her morning walks, Susan was beginning to feel more energetic, although her cough was still present.

Nevertheless, her minor improvement in energy reassured her that she was on the right track. Not all of the people in her life were quite as convinced, though. While her husband and three grown children were supportive of her decision not to use conventional medicine, many of her friends were upset with her for making such a bold decision:

> *I was very discriminating about the people I surrounded myself with. Because I chose not to use any Western medicine methods, I had a number of friends who really isolated themselves from me. They moved away because they didn't want to see me, because they didn't want to watch me die—those were their words. And I just really didn't want to be around people who were carrying that energy. They were "tracking" my death, and I wasn't. . . . I wanted to be around the highest vibration of frequencies possible.*

So, Susan made sure to surround herself only with people who supported her choices. During this time, she also made a conscious attempt to feel more joy in her life, and one of the ways she achieved this was by "not worrying about the past and not worrying about the future." Instead, she tried to focus on being fully present in each moment, including while she was researching for hours on end at the local library. Her research eventually led her beyond the physical body and into a world that was foreign yet simultaneously fascinating to her, the world of energy medicine, acupuncture meridians, and the concept of energy blockages:

> *I ended up studying Traditional Chinese Medicine in terms of learning the meridian system and how that interacts with the auric field and the chakras. . . . I'd never been involved in any of this! And then I actually went to a five-day training with Donna*

Eden and started using a lot of the techniques that Donna uses to trace meridians to get energy flowing. . . . My best understanding is that when energy is stuck in the body such that it's able to be recorded in a scan such as a PET scan—because that does show hot spots—that Western allopathic medicine doesn't have a way to describe stuck energy. And so their description becomes "a tumor," "a mass," any of those kind of fill-in-the-blanks, because they don't have a way of saying that energy has conscripted or congealed. So, my goal became not so much finding out why *it happened but how to get that energy to move.*

The notion that a cancerous tumor is simply a buildup of stuck energy gave Susan a new, less fearful way of thinking about the diagnosis her doctors had given her. So she started using energy medicine and kinesiology techniques—such as Donna Eden's and Machaelle Small Wright's methods—to learn how to trace the energy in her body and *feel* where it was stuck. This gave Susan a powerful sense of control over her health. She began tracing her energy meridians every day and followed up with energy release exercises designed to get her energy unstuck and flowing again. During my interview with Susan, I asked her if she had any ideas about why her energy had become stuck in her pancreas, to which she replied:

I really just think that energy was stuck. . . . My understanding of the spleen and pancreas is that not only does it metabolize food, it also metabolizes emotions. And I also know that, from my upbringing, I was born into a very strict German Presbyterian family, for whom showing emotion was not very well accepted, and you were to put a smile on your face and pretty much "stuff it." . . . If [the triple warmer meridian] is scanning for threats all the time, if it's on high alert, then it actually weakens the spleen

meridian. I truly believe that all of those things were critical
to my healing and [were] helping me get into a place where I
was reassuring my own physical body that I was safe, in terms
of calming the triple burner meridian on a regular basis so that
I was in a different place. And I can tell you that today I am a
much different person than I was three years ago.

Susan's in-depth knowledge of the meridian system shows just how much she learned about the intricacies of Traditional Chinese Medicine (TCM), although her unique view of TCM was strongly influenced by Donna Eden, an energy healer. Many people think acupuncture is a treatment that is only physical (due to its needles) and energetic (because the needles are designed to stimulate energy). However, as Susan discovered in her studies, TCM also offers intricate theories on how emotions interact with the physical body. For example, in Donna Eden's view, the energy pathway or "meridian" TCM refers to as the "triple warmer" is known for processing emotions related to feeling safe and protected. So, in Susan's healing work, part of unblocking her "stuck" energy meant cultivating a strong sense of emotional safety and unguardedness.

Another part of Susan's emotional unblocking work had to do with her job and career. Before she came down with her cough, she had an exciting job at a company that sponsored early childhood education programs. As the manager of a new pilot program there, she felt empowered by her position, appreciated its positive contribution to society, and enjoyed the travel that was sometimes required. However, the pilot project—and therefore her job— eventually came to an end, at which point her intuition told her to move on to something new. However, her financial fears led her to accept a different position in the company, one that involved working alone in her home office managing databases:

As I look at it now, the contract [for that pilot project] ended and it really was time for me to leave that job and go do something else. Except I didn't heed that call. . . . [In my new position] I was working from a home office, but I was basically managing a lot of data and not people, and I'm very much a people person. So, I was very stifled by that job. That job I actually took on in July, and in August I had the diagnosis. So, that's how quickly that happened. And I kind of feel like that was the wake-up call. The diagnosis was like "Okay, we tried to tell you that you were supposed to leave and do something else, and you didn't listen."

After her diagnosis, Susan cut back to working part-time for a short while, but as her healing journey deepened and she learned more about the importance of unblocking stuck energy, she eventually realized that she needed to quit her job entirely, which she finally did in March of 2008. Doing this gave her the courage she needed to clear out even more stressful things in her life. For instance, she had spent most of her life caring for other people, such as her children, her husband, her aging parents, or her friends. In fact, her parents raised her to believe that taking care of others was her primary role in life. However, now that healing cancer was her primary role, Susan decided to cut back on some of her caregiving obligations and finally give herself some much-needed "me" time.

At this point, she was single-mindedly focused on clearing away anything that was stuck or no longer serving her. She saw a chiropractor, who was very helpful in releasing stuck energy in her spine. She also got trained in an energy healing technique called Matrix Energetics, which uses the principles of quantum physics, gentle physical touch, and a healing intention to determine where energy is stuck in the body and then to release that stuck energy. Susan describes the subtle technique in this way:

I guess the most basic way of describing [Matrix Energetics] is that, in quantum physics, something can appear as a particle or a wave. . . . And as soon as you have the two points [of the wave], the wave collapses to a particle. What that does is it dispels duality and brings [the wave] back into balance. . . . So, [in Matrix Energetics] you're tracking [your body] to find the two ends of the wave [for a particular problem].

In other words, Susan believes that everything in this world, including our bodies, is made up of vibrating energy. From a scientific perspective, this is true. Far below the level of cells and bacteria and viruses, we are all made up of trillions of atoms that are indeed vibrating at the atomic level.[10] The question, however, is whether using an energy healing technique like Matrix Energetics—which involves using light touch and a healing intention—can actually change the vibration of our atoms enough to lead to a substantial change in our cells. Researchers do not currently have the technology available to test this hypothesis, although many longtime energy healers certainly believe it is possible.

Therefore, I asked Susan whether she thought energy healing could actually lead to physical changes in the body. She described her belief that there is a vibrating field of energy that exists both inside and outside the physical body, called the "energy body" or "etheric body." The energy itself is called "chi," "qi," or "prana" in different healing systems. The physical body is also thought to be made up of energy, although this energy is thought to be vibrating at a much slower frequency, which makes it feel more physically solid (just as H_2O can be in the form of steam, water, or ice). More specifically, she believes that once this energy is inside the body, it uses a system of centers (chakras) and pathways (meridians) to circulate energy around the physical body in order to keep the body operating healthfully. For Susan and most energy healing practitioners, thoughts and emotions exist first and foremost in the energy body. However, because the energy body also penetrates the physical body, they believe repetitive thoughts and emotions can eventually lead to physical blockages in the body, which can eventually lead to disease. Susan explains:

> *I think the etheric body—the energy body—organizes the physical body based on thoughts or emotions that are either flowing or blocked. So, as long as emotions and thoughts are positive and flowing, constantly moving the way that energy is supposed to go, then the physical body is holding a state of greater balance. As soon as the thoughts become low-frequency thoughts, or our emotions become low-frequency emotions, then the energy tends to jam up or get blocked in the energy field. . . . When nothing is done to release those emotions or thoughts, or to change them, then the way that the universe or God or Creator or whatever you call it—the way that "it" can best get your attention is to move those patterns, that stuck energy, closer and closer to the physical body . . . and sometimes even* into *the physical body. And that's what causes what I call "dis-ease." And again, it's still just energy that's stuck and needs to be moved.*

In other words, Susan not only believes that the mind and body are made up of the same substance—energy—but also that certain emotional patterns can lead to that energy getting stuck in the physical body, thereby causing illness. Her theory is quite different from Western medicine, which views illness as something purely physical. In Western medicine, physical organisms such as bacteria or viruses enter the physical body when they are not supposed to, causing problems that lead to disease. Therefore, the Western medicine solution is to remove these physical invaders through physical interventions, such as surgery or medication. In contrast, Susan believes that "dis-ease" is merely stuck energy that often starts getting stuck due to repetitive thought patterns or low-frequency emotions, and over a long enough period of time, that stuck energy turns into a physical blockage or illness. I asked Susan if she believed her cancer was caused by such repetitive thought patterns. She replied:

> *I believe very much that the diagnosis of cancer—or the energy*
> *that was stuck in my body that appeared to be a mass or a tumor*
> *and which my doctors called "cancer"—was caused by these*
> *patterns that I was describing to you that don't get released,*
> *that are continually overlaid, over and over and over, wherever*
> *they are. So, if it's kidney cancer, it's probably excessive fears; if*
> *it's lung cancer, it's grief of some sort that hasn't been resolved.*
> *I think they can be very much tracked back to thought patterns*
> *that are not releasing and therefore they hold in the cell memory.*

Susan's response is based on her studies of Traditional Chinese Medicine, which views each organ as responsible for processing a particular emotion (e.g., the kidneys process fear, and the lungs process grief). One of the most common, repetitive thought patterns cancer patients struggle with is the fear of death. Therefore, when I asked Susan whether she had a fear of death during her healing process, she replied:

> *I think the death of the physical body is simply that. I think that*
> *the death of who we are, the essence of who we are—our soul,*
> *if you call it that—that that doesn't happen, that that goes on.*
> *There's no real death. The only death is a physical death or a*
> *death of this shell, this physical body that we have.*

Susan's belief, similar to that of most religions, is that the soul is the primary aspect of a human being, while the physical body is just the vessel in which the soul temporarily resides. However, she added that if the body is not properly cared for, then it (the body) can die much sooner than it normally would. Susan went on to say that hearing her inner voice say "Not this way, not this time" helped take away her fear of death tremendously, because she suddenly felt taken care of by something larger. During our interview, I asked Susan what or whom she thought the voice might have been. After taking a moment to think, she replied:

> I wish I could say that [the voice I heard] was a guide or a spirit or my higher power, but I think all of those are one and the same. . . . I believe that we are divine beings in physical bodies, that we are more spiritual in nature than we are anything else. However, because we're in human physical bodies, our role is to function on a human level, and so we need both divine energy and human energy—or energy from Mother Earth—in order to stay in balance. But because humans have free will, they choose things—people, emotions, food, all of that—other than that [which] would keep them in balance.

Interestingly, Susan's beliefs about spirituality and divine energy developed as a result of her healing journey and the in-depth studies she engaged in to help herself heal; before then, she had not thought much about such topics. Thanks to her thorough research on how to best care for her vessel of a human body, after about six months of working on healing all the different areas of her life, her cough finally went away. This, more than anything, was a confirmation that she was on the right track. A few months later, her rib pain also disappeared.

As Susan started to feel better, she realized she did not wish to return to her conventional medicine doctors. After all, she had intuitively chosen to use other methods to heal, and she knew that nothing they could say to her now would convince her to stop doing what she was doing. Therefore, she decided she would simply use the disappearance of her symptoms—and the fact that she was still alive after one year—as indicators that the cancer was gone.

It's now been over five years since she received a diagnosis of metastatic pancreatic cancer, and while she has not returned to her doctors and therefore has not definitively confirmed the disappearance of the cancer with Western medicine's scans, her symptoms are gone and she has greatly outlived her doctors' dire prognosis of being dead in less than a year. More important, she feels healthier and happier than ever:

> *I feel great. I love my life—everything! . . . I'm like the classic patient who says "A cancer diagnosis changed my life." . . . I know that that's the whole reason that I called that disease to me: so I could change. . . . The diagnosis was simply an opportunity for me to kind of take a step back, look at life differently, and say, "Okay, what's next?" . . . As I understand it, nothing that happens in our life is a mistake. Everything is a choice, and sometimes we make a choice that takes us down the long and circuitous route, and sometimes we're able to go down the straight and narrow.*

Whether circuitous or straight, Susan's choice to follow her intuition and try alternative healing methods certainly led her back to a place of health. Nowadays, as an avocation, she helps other people, including some with cancer diagnoses, find their own unique paths of healing by encouraging them to follow their intuition and teaching them how to find areas of stuck energy in their bodies:

I've been teaching some free energy classes with the intent of just giving people information that says there are alternatives, there are other options, and you can do a lot for yourself. I try to teach my clients that dying is just one option. . . . So, I give them a visual of the rays of sunshine that come over the horizon at the first moment that the sun bursts over, and that there are as many possibilities of what could happen as there are rays of sunshine. So, you have to pick one that you like and then follow that one.

As you may have guessed, when her clients are unsure about which ray of sunshine to pick, Susan advises them simply to listen to their intuition.

While intuition alone did not heal Susan, it did guide her to various healing modalities that, in her opinion, did heal the cancer. But throughout it all, it was always her inner voice of intuition that guided her along her path.

Action Steps

If you would like to get in touch with your intuition, or strengthen your existing connection to your intuition, here are some simple suggestions to get you started:

- Set aside a time to relax daily while you purposefully let your thinking mind turn off. During this time, don't watch TV or read anything; instead, listen to some calming music and try to let your mind daydream, as opposed to worry or make mental lists.

- Once you are in a relaxed state and your thinking mind has settled down somewhat, choose a technique that allows you to get in touch with the limbic part of your brain, which transmits your intuition. Here are some popular techniques, although you may find your own unique way to access your intuition:

Guided Imagery. There are many guided imagery CDs designed to help you understand a particular issue in your life, such as a medical issue. Download some choices from iTunes or borrow a few CDs from your local library (some of my favorites include those by Belleruth Naparstek and Martin Rossman).

Meditation. Many people have their strongest intuitive insights during meditation. You can start with guided meditation CDs and then eventually wean yourself off the CDs to meditate silently.

Journaling. Some people successfully access the intuitive part of their brains through carefully selected journal prompts, such as "What is the one thing that, if it were to change in my life, would change everything for the better?" or "What are the root causes of this problem?"

Dreams. If you would like to try to access your intuition via dreams, first get into a relaxed state before you fall asleep, and then write an important question on a piece of paper next to your bed. Read it right before you fall asleep, and ask your intuitive self to give you the answer in your dreams. When you awake the next morning, immediately write down as much of your dreams as you can remember, without trying to analyze them. Once you have fully written them down, you can begin to analyze them for intuitive insights.

AS A FRATERNAL twin, I am very familiar with the concept of intuition. I will often randomly start thinking about my twin sister a few seconds before she calls, and there have been times when I have correctly sensed that she was upset, even though we live a thousand miles apart. This kind of intuition is not just limited to twins. I know of best friends, mothers and daughters, and grandparents and grandchildren who are so tightly bonded that they intuitively know how the other person is doing. The Radical Remission survivors in this chapter show us that we can also have that kind of intuitive relationship with our bodies, and listening to such intuition can guide us toward making the changes our bodies are asking us to make in order to regain our health.

That's why, when I am counseling cancer patients, I ask them to go home, get into a relaxed state, and ask their deepest, most intuitive selves these two questions: "What has contributed to my illness?" and "What do my body, mind, and soul need in order to get well again?" I am always amazed by the diversity of answers I hear. Some people say their intuition told them that pesticides on their lawn contributed to their cancer, while others say the death of their mother did. For some people, their intuition tells them they need to move out of a moldy house in order to help the healing process, while others hear they need to forgive their ex-husbands. Regardless of what they hear in answer to these questions, I encourage them to try not to disregard what comes up, even if it doesn't make sense to them right away. After all, we have learned in this chapter that our gut instinct is often right long before our logical mind can explain *why* it is right.

CHAPTER 4

USING HERBS AND SUPPLEMENTS

The art of healing comes from nature, not from the physician.
—PARACELSUS, SIXTEENTH-CENTURY PHYSICIAN

The main difference between chemotherapy and vitamin or herbal supplements is that most chemotherapy is designed to kill cancer cells, while most supplements are designed to strengthen the immune system so that *it* can then remove cancer cells. These two treatment styles stem from two very different belief systems about cancer in general. Today's conventional medicine tends to view cancer as a hostile invader that the body cannot fight off. As a result, outside interventions, such as chemotherapy or radiation, are thought to be necessary. In contrast, many of the alternative healers I interview see cancer as something the body *can* fight off, as long as the body-mind-spirit system is in optimal condition. So, where the typical approach of a conventional oncologist would be to kill cancer cells, the typical approach of an alternative healer would be to strengthen the patient's body-mind-spirit system as much as possible. One of the many ways healers accomplish this is by recommending plant-based herbs and supplements that boost their patients' immune systems. The hope is that, by creating an internal environment that is incredibly strong and healthy, cancer cells will not be able to thrive.

In this chapter, we will look at the two main reasons why Radical Remission survivors take supplements, along with two important caveats to keep in mind when it comes to using supplements. After discussing the research behind herbs and supplements, we'll explore the healing story of a Radical Remission survivor who used supplements to help turn around her non-Hodgkin's lymphoma. At the end of this chapter, I list the most common types of supplements taken by Radical Remission survivors, so that you can, if you wish, begin discussing them with your doctor or nutritionist.

STRENGTHENING THE IMMUNE SYSTEM

By far, the most popular reason I've heard for why Radical Remission survivors and alternative healers recommend taking vitamin and herbal supplements is to strengthen the body's own immune system so it can better find and remove cancer cells from the body. This goes along with an underlying belief that most of my research subjects shared, which is, "To get rid of cancer, you must change the conditions under which it thrives." In other words, they believe cancer can grow and survive only in a certain environment, such as one that is blocked with stagnant energy, lacking in oxygen and nutrients, filled with bacteria and viruses, and so on. Therefore, if you change the underlying conditions of the body, so those conditions become healthier, cancer cells will naturally die off.

The analogy I like to use is a moldy basement. Imagine going into your basement and finding mold everywhere, just as a surgeon sometimes opens up a person's body, only to find cancer everywhere. One strategy to get rid of the mold is to bleach the entire basement, which will certainly kill the mold. This is similar to chemotherapy and radiation, which are both strong interventions that directly kill cancer cells. To continue the analogy, imagine that the bleach has worked and there is now no more mold left in your basement—or no more cancer left in your body. Now your doctor says that all you can do is hope it never comes back.

The issue with this scenario is that the mold in your basement is *destined* to grow back as long as the conditions under which mold thrives—such as darkness and dampness—are still present. However, if you were to bring UV lights into your basement and constantly run a fan and dehumidifier, then the mold would not grow back. This is the main idea behind "changing the conditions under which cancer thrives," and you will notice that all nine factors in this book work toward that goal. The only catch is that the changes must be permanent, otherwise the minute you stop the fan, dehumidifier, or UV light, the old conditions will return and mold may once again grow. That is why the radical survivors I study make mostly permanent changes to their lifestyles, in the hope that they will prevent cancer from ever growing again in their bodies.

One herbalist in Japan tries to change the conditions under which cancer thrives by giving a sharp boost to his cancer patients' immune systems. He does this by placing warm herbs directly on a patient's skin, although only for thirty minutes at a time. First, he forms tiny cones made of charcoal mixed with the herb mugwort (also known as moxa), and then he places these cones in rows along either side of the patient's spine. Once placed, he ignites each cone with a lighter, so the charcoal can warm both the herb and the skin, thereby allowing for more absorption:

[Via a translator:] [The cone] is charcoal and moxa together. When [the herbalist] uses charcoal, he can use it [for a] long time—that's why he uses charcoal. . . . And this [translator holds

up a bottle of liquid vitamin supplement] includes vitamin B17.
He puts it on the skin before he puts on the moxa. . . . He says this
[entire herbal treatment] makes the immune system stronger. It
makes new cells.

Moxa, or mugwort, is a popular herb in Traditional Chinese Medicine, known for its ability to stimulate the circulation of blood and chi (i.e., life-force energy). It is best absorbed through the skin when it is hot, which is why the herb is traditionally burned and then held close to the skin. However, this Japanese herbalist enhances the traditional moxa treatment by adding liquid vitamin B17, also known as laetrile, a powerful, immune-boosting nutrient our ancestors used to get from eating millet, sorghum, and certain other foods but is now virtually nonexistent in the Standard American Diet.

Similar to this Japanese herbalist, "Brendan" is a gastric cancer survivor who also uses herbs and supplements to strengthen his immune system. He refused all conventional medicine treatment after he was diagnosed with advanced stomach cancer at the age of forty-eight; he simply figured his "time was up" and therefore did not want to suffer through the painful side effects of chemotherapy and surgery. His doctors told him if he refused treatment, he would not live to see the new year. Nevertheless, he had watched too many friends suffer terribly from the effects of cancer treatment, only to die in the end, so he held firm to his decision. However, he did begin reading about alternative approaches to treatment, and this eventually led him to take a wide variety of vitamin and herbal supplements:

Dr. William Donald Kelley's research made a lot of sense to me,
where he treats cancer as a type of placenta sack that shows up in

the wrong spot. His treatment involves basically telling the body— chemically—to have an abortion. So, I started following Kelley's procedures and got myself on IP-6 [a vitamin supplement]. . . . Since IP-6 is the messenger molecule, it needs a message to carry, and that is made of trace minerals. So, I added a trace mineral supplement. But the molecule is still considered a free radical by the body, so I added vitamin C to allow free radical passage from the bloodstream through the cell walls. Then [I added] aloe vera juice [and] vitamin E, to aid in cell reproduction and recovery. Add to that the arid climate of the West [because he moved from the East Coast to the western United States] and eliminating the reinfection of flukes and parasites—well, my immune system returned to being able to do what it was designed to do, without being overwhelmed. I added some antiparasite herbs and, come Thanksgiving, was doing quite well.

Finding this complex combination of supplements turned out to be what Brendan's particular body needed to boost his immune system in such a way that it was able to identify and remove the cancerous cells in his stomach. Six years later (and counting), he remains cancer-free and has stayed on a modified supplement regimen.

DETOXIFYING THE BODY

The second reason Radical Remission survivors choose to take vitamin and herbal supplements is to clear the body of toxins, such as pesticides, chemicals, heavy metals, bacteria, viruses, and parasites. While in many ways our world is cleaner than it has ever been, advances in technology have also replaced simple germs and bacteria with things like chemically engineered pesticides, heavy metals, and antibiotic-resistant bacteria. Many of the healers and survivors I study believe that these complex chemicals, which are now ever-present in our environment, send confusing messages to the body, leading to dysregulation at best and disease at worst.

One healer who believes cancer patients need to detoxify their bodies of any lingering bacteria and viruses is a man named Dr. Katsunari Nishihara from Japan. Dr. Nishihara has a theory that there is no such thing as an autoimmune disease. Rather, he believes that diseases such as arthritis, lupus, and even cancer are the result of bacteria and viruses that have infiltrated healthy cells. Therefore, what may look like the body incorrectly attacking itself (as in the case of autoimmune diseases) or what may look like cells suddenly going "crazy" as they replicate uncontrollably (in the case of cancer) is, in Dr. Nishihara's opinion, an indication that cells have been infected with either a bacteria or a virus. According to his theory, the body sometimes recognizes this infiltration and therefore tries to attack the infected cells, which is what we see happening in auto-immune diseases when the body attacks itself. However, sometimes bacteria or viruses are very skilled at hiding within cells (i.e., putting up chemical masks), and therefore the immune system walks right past them. We know this is what happens with the HIV virus, and Dr. Nishihara believes this is also what happens with cancer.

Dr. Nishihara's theory has some merit to it, as scientists already know that the *H. pylori* bacteria leads to stomach cancer and the human papillomavirus (HPV) leads to uterine cancer. Therefore, it is not so extreme to think that other bacteria and viruses might lead to other cancers; in fact, many scientists already agree with Dr. Nishihara on this point.[1] What is most interesting to me, however, is the way in which he uses this theory to guide his treatment of cancer patients.

He believes that a slightly low core body temperature—which

is usually measured by a rectal thermometer and can be caused by either stress or lack of movement (e.g., sitting at a computer all day)—weakens our cells by damaging their mitochondria. This opens the door for bacteria and viruses to infiltrate the cell and cause it to become cancerous. More specifically, Dr. Nishihara believes that, in the case of cancer, bacteria that are supposed to stay confined to the digestive tract (called enterobacteria) find a way to migrate outside the intestinal walls and infect mitochondria-damaged cells elsewhere in the body.

As a result of this theory, Dr. Nishihara works backward: He first treats the infection in the cells by prescribing specific antibiotics or antivirals that are tailored to each cancer patient. Next, to keep the digestive tract as free of bacteria and viruses as possible, he prescribes a special prebiotic supplement that contains bifidus factor, which is a substance that promotes the growth of healthy intestinal flora. He describes this supplement:

> *[I recommend] having bifidus factor after every meal. It's for the enterobacteria. If we have such bifidus factor, the intestine inside becomes very nice [healthy]. . . . Bifidus factor means the cultured medium of* Bacillus bifidum. *[After] many kinds of culturing, and after boiling and killing all the bacterium, almost all of [the] core enzymes and vitamins and minerals for* Bacillus bifidum *are growing very nice [healthfully]—this is bifidus factor. . . . Chlorella—do you know it? Green foods. They are also quite similar to bifidus factor.*

After prescribing this important prebiotic supplement, Dr. Nishihara tries to prevent the cancer from recurring by repairing the mitochondria in his patients' cells. To achieve this, he tries to raise their core body temperature by recommending they eat only hot foods, drink only warm liquids, practice deep breathing, reduce their stress, exercise regularly, and get plenty of sleep and sunlight. Dr. Nishihara also recommends that his patients breathe as much as possible through their noses, because he believes the nose is better at preventing bacteria from entering the body than the mouth is. With this multifaceted treatment approach, including the important supplement of bifidus factor to help detoxify the body, Dr. Nishihara has helped many of his cancer patients have Radical Remissions.

SUPPLEMENTS ALONE MAY NOT BE ENOUGH

While the participants in my research laud the benefits of supplements to help a sick body regain balance and health, they are also quick to note that one should not rely on supplements as magic bullets. Unfortunately, Americans in general have grown quite passive about taking care of their bodies. Many people think they can treat their bodies however they want and then simply take a pill when things start to go wrong. For instance, when their blood pressure is high, they think first to take a pill instead of reducing their stress and increasing their sleep. When their back chronically aches, they think first to pop a pain pill instead of reducing the amount of time they spend sitting in a chair during the day and increasing the amount of exercise they do each week.

Similarly, the solution to cancer is not only to take supplements. Supplements certainly have a place; they make up for vital nutrients and minerals not often found in today's food supply, and they help the body detoxify the chemicals from our modern environment. Nevertheless, they are not the single solution.

One Radical Remission survivor who feels strongly about this is a natural healing advocate named Chris Wark. At only twenty-six years old, Chris was shocked to be diagnosed with stage 3 colon cancer and was immediately rushed into surgery. Although the surgery successfully removed a large tumor from his colon, his doctors still insisted on chemotherapy because the cancer had also spread to his lymph nodes. Much to their dismay, Chris refused the chemotherapy, saying that he first wanted to try more natural methods of healing. His doctors told him he was "insane."

Nevertheless, Chris went forward with this plan and radically changed his diet along the lines of what we saw in chapter 1. He then looked for someone to advise him on which supplements to take, which led him to clinical nutritionist John Smothers at the Integrative Wellness and Research Center in Memphis, Tennessee. John was the first person to tell Chris that he had done the right thing by refusing chemo and, instead, changing his diet and lifestyle, and this made John an instant ally and friend. Chris describes his supplement use this way:

Along with a strict anticancer diet, my nutritionist recommended many different nutraceutical-grade herbal supplements to address issues common to all cancer patients: liver detoxification, Candida/fungal overgrowth, parasites, suppressed immune function, and nutritional deficiencies. However, a radical change of diet and lifestyle is foundational to healing; supplements are "supplemental." The right supplements can provide additional support to the healing functions in the body, but if you are not willing to make necessary changes to your diet and lifestyle, supplements won't do you much good. In other words, if you keep eating processed food, drinking beer, smoking cigarettes, and not moving your body, you are not likely to see much benefit from supplements. Taking supplements without a radical change of diet and lifestyle is like fighting a house fire with a squirt gun.

Less than a year after his diagnosis Chris was declared cancer-free, and things have stayed that way since 2004. His doctors were and continue to be baffled, but Chris is not; he is convinced that the major changes he made in terms of diet, lifestyle, and supplements were what led to his healing.

DIET ALONE MAY NOT BE ENOUGH

While supplements by themselves may not lead to Radical Remission, many of the people I research found that supplements were the missing link they had been searching for in their healing journeys. For example, many started out by radically changing their diets, yet their cancer did not fully go away, or else the cancer came back. For these people, it wasn't until they added certain supplements—and the exact supplements vary from person to person—that their bodies finally received all the nutrients and minerals they needed to fully remove their cancer.

One such Radical Remission survivor is Ann Fonfa. After being diagnosed with breast cancer at age forty-four, Ann had a lumpectomy but refused chemotherapy and radiation because she was extremely chemically sensitive at the time. Her cancer unfortunately returned some months after the lumpectomy, and over the next few years she was on a roller coaster of surgery, followed by a brief remission, followed by a recurrence, followed by another surgery. In total, she underwent two more lumpectomies, a left mastectomy, and eventually a right mastectomy, but chemo and radiation were never possible due to her extreme chemical sensitivity. Feeling like she had no choice but to look for other options, Ann began exploring complementary medicine, and her journey led her to make major changes in her diet, exercise regimen, and stress management. Five years after her initial diagnosis, Ann was still alive, even though her tumors kept stubbornly growing back. That's when she visited a Chinese herbalist in New York City named Dr. George Wong:

[Dr. Wong] suggested that I start taking his herbs and cease taking all of the dietary supplements that I knew had kept me alive, causing each tumor to grow slower than the last—even slower than normal cells. We finally agreed that I would take his herbs in addition *to my supplements. My whole body was covered in hives after drinking the first tea. After the hives went away, though, it quickly became clear that the multiple chemical sensitivity I suffered from—which had caused me to refuse chemo and radiation treatments—had reduced in intensity. . . . I was much better. I continued with the herbs, and with all of my other lifestyle changes, and never had a tumor again.*

In other words, Ann's other alternative treatments—diet change, exercise, stress management, and vitamin supplements—had helped keep her cancer in check for five years, but it wasn't until she took the additional supplement of Chinese herbs that her immune system was finally able to eradicate her cancer completely. Ann has been cancer-free for over fourteen years, and she now dedicates her life to the Annie Appleseed Project, a nonprofit organization that provides free information to cancer patients about complementary cancer therapies.

THE SCIENCE BEHIND HERBS AND SUPPLEMENTS

Ideally, we would get all the vitamins and minerals our immune systems need from diet alone. However, this is sadly not as possible today as it was a hundred years ago, due to the current practices of corporate farming. To begin with, today's fruits and vegetables lack important trace minerals. That's because pesticides and modern farming practices strip minerals from the soil. To make up for this, corporate farmers artificially add minerals back into the soil; however, they typically add back in only the three major ones: nitrogen, phosphorus, and potassium (N-P-K). They do not add back in trace minerals, which scientists have only recently realized are essential for the functioning of our immune systems.[2]

In addition to this lack of trace minerals, today's fruits and vegetables contain much smaller amounts of vitamins than they did a hundred years ago. This is due to pesticide use, the same lack of trace minerals in the soil, and the harvesting of fruits and vegetables long before they are ripe in order to transport them across the country. Consider this staggering fact: today's fruits and vegetables have up to 40 percent fewer vitamins and minerals than they did just fifty years ago.[3] Some studies have shown that eating organic fruits and vegetables can help make up for this nutrient deficiency,[4] while other studies have found that there is not much difference in nutrient content between conventional and organic produce. (However, these same studies show that organic foods do contain significantly fewer pesticides than conventionally grown food.[5]) Given this widespread lack of minerals and nutrients in the food supply, you can see why supplements may be necessary for maintaining health in today's world.

However, when it comes to the science, the jury is still out. Sadly, this is because many herbal supplements cannot be patented, and therefore large pharmaceutical companies have very little incentive to conduct research on them—because they would not be able to make money off them. This leaves only governmental and private institutions to fund studies on vitamins and herbs, which explains why there have been so few large, long-term studies that look at supplements and cancer.

Nevertheless, smaller studies have shown that various supplements do indeed have cancer-fighting properties. For example, numerous studies done on epigallocatechin gallate (ECGC)—a compound found in green tea—have found that it actively kills cancer cells,[6] while other studies have found that mushroom supplements such as "turkey tail" increase the number of natural killer cells in cancer patients.[7] Additional studies have shown that high doses of vitamin C,[8] high doses of turmeric spice,[9] and daily doses of probiotics[10] all help boost the immune system's cancer-fighting capabilities. This is only a small sampling of studies that have been done on the wide variety of supplements used for cancer. The majority of the studies, while small, nevertheless show that supplements provide minor to significant benefits to the body, which is promising given the fact that these supplements often have few, if any, side effects.

While we are still a long way from seeing the results of many large, multiyear, million-dollar studies on supplement use, a few large studies have been conducted. One such study, published in the *Journal of the American Medical Association* (*JAMA*), followed 14,600 men over fourteen years and found that those who took a daily multivitamin ended up reducing their risk of cancer slightly.[11] This study is an important first step in what will hopefully be more large-scale studies looking at the effectiveness of supplement use on cancer. In the meantime, Radical Remission survivors tend to agree with the advice of a report from *JAMA,* which stated, "Most people do not consume an optimal amount of all vitamins by diet alone. . . . It appears prudent for all adults to take vitamin supplements."[12]

———

NOW THAT WE have covered the main reasons Radical Remission survivors choose to take supplements, I invite you to immerse yourself in the healing story of "Jenny," a Radical Remission survivor who used all of this book's nine key factors, but especially herbs and supplements, to overcome her rare form of non-Hodgkin's lymphoma.

—⌘ Jenny's Story ⌘—

Jenny enjoyed fifty-one wonderful years of life, which included a loving husband, three amazing children, and a successful small business, before she heard the words "You have cancer." Then in May of 2008, while preparing for a minor, elective surgery, her slightly abnormal blood test results led her doctor to discover that she actually had advanced follicular lymphoma, also called non-Hodgkin's lymphoma. This was despite the fact that she felt perfectly normal and had no noticeable symptoms. Once the diagnosis was confirmed by a bone marrow biopsy, panic and fear sank heavily into both Jenny's and her husband's stomachs. In fact, they could not even talk to each other without one of them starting to cry. In spite of this inevitable fear, which goes along with any cancer diagnosis, Jenny did not want to live the rest of her life feeling scared and sad, so she soon decided that cancer was going to have to be on board with *her,* and not the other way around. She would somehow find a way to manage her cancer, because dying was simply not an option in her mind.

While this fierce determination helped reduce Jenny's fear somewhat, her first meeting with her oncologist did not:

In the very beginning, I was basically lied to by my oncologist.
He told me, "You have cancer, but don't worry. I can cure
this one. And we're going to put you on CHOP-R [a multiple-
drug chemotherapy regimen]." I was so floored. I mean, I was
asymptomatic! I had no symptoms. . . . I felt like I got sucker

punched. And I was going to do the chemotherapy, but in the meantime, I started googling my disease and I started learning that my disease is not curable. So, the fact that he said that to me made me uneasy. And then I went and [requested a copy of] my medical records, and I found out that there were a couple of other things that he was not being completely truthful with me about.

For example, in her medical records, Jenny's doctor had written down that he had offered her three different types of chemotherapy and that among those she had chosen CHOP-R, a five-drug chemotherapy cocktail consisting of cyclophosphamide, hydroxydaunorubicin, vincristine (brand name Oncovin), prednisone, and rituximab. Her doctor had never mentioned any option other than CHOP-R, and even if he *had* offered her a choice, she would have had no idea which one to choose. This was all before she had even had a PET scan, which was something she had learned from her online research was very important:

[My oncologist] had my bone marrow biopsy and I said to him, "But what about the PET scan?" And he goes, "That's not necessary. We don't really need it." And I said, "I would really like to have a PET scan to confirm what you've found," because the two kind of confirm each other, right? And plus, the bone marrow biopsy was not conclusive. The pathologist said [in his report], "We believe that this is follicular lymphoma, but it could be splenic marginal zone [lymphoma]." And I asked [my oncologist] what that meant. He had never brought that to my attention, but because I pulled my medical records, I found out. And so I asked him and he said, "Oh, it doesn't mean anything. You have non-Hodgkin's lymphoma and this is the treatment that we're going to do."

In other words, the pathologist who had analyzed her bone marrow under a microscope could tell for sure that she had non-Hodgkin's lymphoma, but he could not tell for sure which *type* she had. There are many different types of non-Hodgkin's lymphoma, and Jenny had learned from her online research that different types require different treatments. That is why she wanted to have a PET scan, to help determine which type of lymphoma she had. Despite her doctor's annoyance, Jenny insisted on having a PET scan before she started the CHOP-R—and thank goodness she did. The PET scan showed large amounts of cancer in her spleen, which was very enlarged—it was sixteen centimeters wide and holding approximately eight pounds of cancer. This combined with the fact that the PET scan showed no enlarged lymph nodes anywhere else in her body strongly indicated that Jenny had splenic marginal zone lymphoma, not follicular lymphoma.

Despite all of this, Jenny's doctor, who by now was quite annoyed with her, told her that it still did not matter because the treatment would be the same for either type of lymphoma: CHOP-R. At this point, Jenny's intuition told her to do a little more research before following this doctor's treatment plan. So, she spent five thousand dollars of her personal savings to get a second opinion from a different hospital:

After I took my bone marrow biopsy to [a different hospital], I found out that the treatment is not *the same, that with splenic marginal zone [lymphoma] the very first treatment they would start out with would be the "R" [rituximab] only. They would leave the "CHOP" out. And that's* huge *for the fact that that's four different drugs that I would not have to deal with in my body—hydroxydaunorubicin being one of them, which damages the heart, and another one which causes secondary cancer. I could actually bypass those and only use the rituximab. But [my doctor] wasn't offering me any other choices. He was telling me we were going to do CHOP-R.*

Jenny then spent an additional five thousand dollars of her personal savings to get a third opinion at yet another hospital. This third hospital agreed that all signs were pointing to splenic marginal zone lymphoma, which is a much more slow-growing cancer than follicular lymphoma. They even said that she could "watch and wait" for a few months instead of jumping in with the rituximab. Hearing this gave Jenny a surge of relief, because she suddenly felt like she had more time to deal with her cancer. It also made her realize that she absolutely had to find a way to switch to a new oncologist. However, her health insurance was part of a health management organization (HMO), which made it difficult for her to switch doctors even within her HMO, and it was impossible for her to see doctors at outside hospitals.

As quietly as she could, Jenny put in a request to switch to a different oncologist within her HMO. Unfortunately, she was assigned to a very young doctor who was brand new to oncology. She liked the fact that he did not argue with her when she told him via a telephone call that she wanted to follow the watch-and-wait protocol recommended by the third hospital. During her first in-person appointment with him, however, her confidence plummeted:

The doctor came in and said, "How are we doing today?" I said, "Good." He said, "Okay, I'll see you back in three months." And then he was leaving! And I said to him, "What do you do during 'wait and watch'?" He said, "Well, we check your stats"—because they pull your blood three days before you go in—"and then we feel and make sure there's no more enlarged lymph nodes." And

I said, "Well, what part of that did we do today?"—because he
hadn't even opened up the computer! And he said, "Why?" And I
said, "Because I pulled my test results on my blood and they're not
looking so good right now." And he said, "Really?" And he ran right
over and opened up his computer. . . . And that's when I decided
he was not going to be a team member for me.

At this point, Jenny had learned the importance of immediately
requesting a copy of all her lab results—which is the right of any
patient—and she was becoming adept at interpreting them. (Personally, I think this can be a wonderful practice for people who wish to
take a more active role in their health, although the final interpretation of any results should always be done by a doctor.) Meanwhile,
she was worried because she could feel her spleen getting larger by the
week. So, she switched to yet another oncologist within her HMO,
and this one was thankfully more experienced and more open to
the idea of watchful waiting. However, he was very concerned about
Jenny's spleen rupturing. Even riding in a car was dangerous, he said,
because a sudden jolt could cause her seat belt to rupture her spleen.
This news frightened her immensely, so she asked if having surgery
to remove the spleen was a possibility, to which he replied, "If that's
what you'd like, we'll do it." However, the surgeon to whom he then
referred her disagreed, saying that removing her spleen would only
make her lymphoma spread faster to her bone marrow.

By now, Jenny was feeling thoroughly confused, afraid, and dis-
trustful of anyone in the medical system. After further consultation
with the doctors from the third hospital, she decided she would not
do the surgery or take the rituximab but instead would try to deal
with her enlarged spleen using more natural methods. For example,
the oncologist she had seen at the third hospital had suggested that
changing her eating habits might boost her immune system:

[The doctor at the third hospital] told me and my husband, "I think that if you change your diet and stop eating 'dead' food and start eating 'live' food, and if you supplement and you juice [vegetables and fruits], I think you could probably manage this disease very nicely for years before you have to do any chemotherapy." . . . So, I had to make a decision about whether or not I was going to build my immune system to try to fight [my cancer] or whether I should try to suppress my immune system because my disease is of the immune system. And I chose to build my immune system.

Once Jenny decided she was going to try to build up her immune system, she followed this doctor's advice and completely changed how she ate. Based on the many books and articles she was reading voraciously, as well as the advice of a nutritionist she consulted with, Jenny immediately stopped eating all refined and processed foods, including the frozen, low-calorie meals she had been eating for years. She also started eating mostly raw fruits and vegetables, whole grains, and beans. She bought a juicer, drank fresh vegetable juice in the morning, and ate lots of organic fruits and vegetables throughout the day. She also stopped drinking coffee, switching instead to green tea, and eliminated sugar from her diet almost completely. Based on her research and consultation with the nutritionist, she also began taking a wide variety of supplements at this time:

Systemic enzymes—those are huge [very important]. . . . I take them three times a day on an empty stomach. I also take digestive enzymes, and I take a shiitake-maitake-lychee mushroom [and fruit] mix. And I take grape seed, magnesium, and lysine. I take a [brand name] product that has dandelion, turmeric, and milk thistle. I take selenium. I take [a brand name supplement blend]

*which has cordyseps, lion's mane, and all sorts of stuff that I can't
even pronounce, but it's for immune building. I take zinc. I
take vitamin C, quercetin, bromelain, IP-6, and inositol. And
prebiotics and probiotics. I take a lot!*

While it was neither easy nor cheap for her to take all these
supplements, Jenny still thought it was easier than dealing with the
short- and long-term side effects of chemotherapy. That is not to say
that these supplements did not have any side effects at all. In fact,
one of the most common side effects of a radical diet change or a
new supplementation program is what is known as a "die-off" or
"detox" reaction. This refers to the sudden death of many bacteria
and yeast that were previously able to live in your body before you
began cleaning it out. Sometimes your body has a hard time clearing out such a large, sudden amount of dead bacteria and yeast, so
this can lead to a temporary period of headaches, bloating, chills, or
even a mild fever:

*It was difficult in the beginning, because sometimes with
[systemic enzymes] there can be a huge kill-off, a yeast kill-off,
and it can make your stomach upset. . . . Garlic is also one that's
hard for me to take in supplement form. I can cook with it and
eat it raw in my salsa, but when I take it in pill form, it always
upsets my stomach.*

After a few weeks of dealing with minor die-off symptoms,
such as bloating and headaches, those reactions wore off and Jenny
began to feel more energetic. More important, she also could feel
her spleen beginning to shrink slightly. This helped convince her
that she had made the right decision by refusing the surgery and
chemotherapy, and it also motivated her to keep searching for new

things to try. In her research, she came across an integrative doctor in Nevada who had had good success treating lymphoma patients:

I went to see [the integrative doctor] in Reno, Nevada. He is a Western medicine doctor, but he also deals in alternatives. And he has a lymphoma [supplement] formula. . . . My friend also has splenic marginal zone lymphoma and her insurance pays to see him, so I hitchhiked in with her [accompanied her] on one of her office visits. . . . He has a lymphoma recipe . . . and it's got everything in it. To be honest with you, you spend that much going out and getting everything individually, you really do. It's got all the glandulars in it, it's got quercetin, it's got resveratrol, it's got your vitamins A, C, D, E—it's got it all.

So, Jenny began taking this special lymphoma supplement along with her other supplements and new diet. In addition, she tried to manage her emotional health. For example, when she was first diagnosed she and her husband—who have known each other since they were young and have been married for over thirty years—were both "emotional wrecks." They were so filled with fear regarding her possible early death that they finally reached out for help, first from conventional medicine:

My husband and I finally went and got mood elevators [from their general practitioner], but that was worse! Because then, during the day, you had no emotion, and when it wore off at night, you sank into this huge depression. We did that for three weeks and I looked at him and said, "We can't do this. We have to deal with this!" . . . So, I actually did a lot of meditation. I did a lot of going within myself. I would go to sleep with meditation tapes going, so that that was what I was thinking about when I

slept. I realized that I needed to stop thinking in that [fearful]
direction and think in a more positive way.

In addition to using guided meditation CDs to try to release her
fear and increase her positive emotions, Jenny connected with a
clinical psychologist who specializes in helping cancer patients let
go of any deep-seated, suppressed emotions from their past. Jenny
worked with him over the phone, and during their sessions he
taught her an emotional release technique that involved trying to
recall traumatic events from her past while tapping certain parts of
her body. The tapping is believed to release energetic and emotional
blockages in the body, similar to how acupressure or acupuncture
works. Jenny explains:

> *I started to talk to this one [psychologist] over the phone, and*
> *that's what he concentrates on—going within yourself and getting*
> *rid of all of the negative stuff that's on your heart. I did really*
> *focus on that, but it's much easier said than done . . . because*
> *in life there are a lot of things we can't control. So, whether*
> *negativity comes in and out of your life, you can't control that.*
> *But you do have to learn to try to let it go as much as possible.*

As Jenny purposefully tried to focus on the positive aspects of
her life while also letting go of any negative events from her past
or present, she realized that she still had one major emotional challenge left to face: the fear of death. She had always considered herself to be spiritual, but after her diagnosis, she began having daily
"talks" with God:

> *You really start asking yourself, "What's on the other side?" So, I*
> *definitely had to deal with my spirituality. . . . And now I'm not*

afraid anymore. I'm not afraid one way or the other. I know that
I have to stay right here because I have so much to do, and so that
helps me live, and that helps me heal because I have to [heal].
I have to be here for the people who need me. But on the other
hand, I'm okay if I cross over because I feel that I've been a good
enough human being, that whatever's on the other side, I can go.
So, the fear is gone, and I think that's probably what poisons a
lot of people. You can't be afraid of it [death]. . . . I mean you're
gonna die some time.

After working diligently on her physical, emotional, and spiritual health, Jenny felt that she was in a better emotional place, with fewer lows and more centeredness. She was vigilant about sticking to her mostly raw diet, taking all the supplements she and her nutritionist had chosen to help her body heal, and managing her stress and emotions. She also continued with the same daily exercise regimen she had created for herself years earlier. As the weeks turned into months, she could feel her spleen shrinking more. It eventually got to a point when she could no longer feel her spleen at all from the outside, which is exactly how it should be. And her juicing and supplement routine—although much more time consuming than her previous habit of quickly heating up a frozen meal—was, in her opinion, well worth the effort in terms of the effects on her health:

I probably took—and still take—about forty pills a day. Not all
at once, but throughout the day. I take the prebiotic early, when
I get up, and [then] I take a large amount of [the supplements]
first thing in the morning when my husband juices for me. . . .
You see, overnight you're fasting. So, when you wake up in the
morning, you haven't eaten for eight hours and your body is
hungry. So, what I do is—the first thing in the morning—I take

a good majority of my supplements, with my digestive enzymes,
[and] with my [freshly pressed] juice. And the probiotic goes in
with my juice and my supplements. And I take eighteen systemic
enzymes a day—six of them, three times a day. I like to take those
with magnesium, on an empty stomach. You want to take them
an hour before or after you eat.

With gratitude instead of annoyance, Jenny happily took these forty pills a day, because she could feel the positive effects they were having on her health. Seven months after her initial diagnosis, she was feeling so good that she decided she was ready for a follow-up bone marrow biopsy. To her doctors' complete surprise—but not to Jenny's—the test came back completely negative for any cancerous cells. Unable to believe what they were seeing, they sent her in for a follow-up PET scan. Again to her doctors' amazement, the scan showed that her spleen had returned to a normal size and her entire body had no evidence of any cancer.

It has now been over five years since Jenny was first diagnosed with stage 4 splenic marginal zone lymphoma. Since her diagnosis, she has taken control of her healing by finding the right doctor, radically changing her diet, and taking a host of supplements she believes boosted her immune system so that it could remove her cancer. She is monitored regularly through blood tests, bone marrow biopsies, and PET scans, which all continue to come back clear. Her doctors have written "spontaneous remission" on her medical report. She, of course, knows this because she continues to request copies of all her medical records. However, Jenny strongly disagrees with this word "spontaneous":

I have been diagnosed with spontaneous remission on paper.
However, I do not believe it was from doing nothing. I changed

*almost my entire lifestyle when I got diagnosed . . . and I have
gone all over looking for a doctor to help me with a game
plan. . . . In the past few years I have lost many friends—and
my dad—to the effects of Western medicine for cancer. . . .
Meanwhile, I am still in remission and going strong. I even met
my new grandson last December.*

ONE OF THE most important healing factors for Jenny was finding the right combination of supplements that gave her immune
system the boost it needed to remove cancer fully from her body.
Although the supplements alone would not likely have led to her
remission, the supplements combined with all the other lifestyle
changes she made was the recipe her particular body needed for
healing.

Action Steps

Most of the Radical Remission survivors I study take supplements
that fall into the following three categories. Keep in mind, though,
that just as Jenny spent hours researching on her own and consulting with qualified nutritionists and doctors, you too should do your
own research and find a qualified nutritionist or doctor to help
you choose the supplements that are best suited to your particular
health situation.

Category One: Supplements to Help You Digest Your Food

- *Digestive Enzymes.* These help your digestive system break
  down food. Specific examples include proteolytic enzymes
  and pancreatic enzymes.

• *Prebiotics and Probiotics.* Probiotics are the beneficial or "good" bacteria that live in your digestive tract and help you digest your food and strengthen your immune system. Many people are deficient in probiotics due to our culture's frequent use of antibiotics, which indiscriminately kill all bacteria in your digestive tract, both the good and the bad. Probiotics feed on prebiotics, which is why it is helpful to take both types of supplements.

Category Two: Supplements to Detoxify Your Body

• *Antifungals.* These help reduce *Candida* and other fungi that are often overgrown in most Americans' digestive tracts. Examples of natural antifungals include olive leaf extract, horsetail plant, and stinging nettle.

• *Antiparasitics.* These help reduce parasites that can take root in your digestive tract and interfere with your digestion and immune system. Examples of antiparasitics include black walnut hull, wormwood, and goldenseal.

• *Antibacterials and Antivirals.* These help eliminate any underlying bacterial or viral infections in your body. Examples include garlic, oil of oregano, and pau d'arco.

• *Liver Detoxifiers.* The liver is your primary detoxification organ, and supplements can make its job easier, especially when it comes to removing heavy metals. Examples include milk thistle, dandelion root, and licorice root.

Category Three: Supplements to Boost Your Immune System

• *Immune System Boosters.* Many herbs and vitamins help boost the immune system. Popular ones among Radical Remission survivors are aloe vera, vitamin C, certain mushrooms, fish oil, and trace minerals.

- *Vitamins and Hormones.* Many survivors supplement with vitamin B12, vitamin D, and melatonin until their blood levels of these vitamins and hormones return to within a normal range. You can ask your doctor to test your current levels of these with a simple blood test, and the results will tell you whether or not you need to take supplements.

———

WHILE I PERSONALLY take many of the supplements listed, after studying cancer for over a decade I have come to the conclusion that supplements are merely Band-Aids for a nutrient-poor, toxin-rich environment. While they can certainly help us when we find our bodies riddled with cancer, I do not think they should be considered a long-term solution.

For example, if we started eating how our ancestors ate, we would eat a small amount of fermented food every day, such as homemade kombucha tea or sauerkraut, which would allow us to stop using probiotic supplements. If we cooked with more antibacterial foods and herbs, such as garlic or turmeric, we could cut down on our unrestrained use of antibiotics. If we moved our bodies not just daily but *hourly,* we could stop taking supplements for pain, such as glucosamine. The list goes on: Sleeping for eight or more hours per night in complete darkness would allow us to stop taking supplements like melatonin. Getting fifteen minutes of sun exposure each day would allow us stop taking vitamin D supplements. Eating a diet low in sugar and processed carbohydrates would allow us to stop taking anti-inflammatory supplements such as fish oil or resveratrol. Finally, cutting down on the amount of toxic metals, chemicals, plastics, and electromagnetic radiation we are exposed to each day would allow us to cut down on detoxifying supplements like milk thistle or dandelion root.

Therefore, when I counsel people who want either to prevent or to recover from cancer, I first recommend that they discuss with their doctor the three categories of supplements listed previously to help get their systems back on track. However, once their bodies have returned to a state of balance, I recommend they slowly wean off the supplements while they learn to "supplement" their lives with other things, such as a fruit- and vegetable-filled diet, a windowsill herb garden, homemade kombucha tea, nontoxic cleaning products, a regular bedtime, and a daily exercise routine.

CHAPTER 5

RELEASING SUPPRESSED EMOTIONS

*Anger is an acid that can do more harm to the vessel in which it is
stored than to anything on which it is poured.*

—MARK TWAIN

Surprisingly, only two of the nine most frequent factors of Radical Remission in this book are physical (diet change and herbs/supplements); the rest are emotional or spiritual in nature. When I first started this research, I fully expected the most common things people would report doing for their healing to be physical in nature, such as changing their diets, taking supplements, exercising, having coffee enemas. Therefore, no one was more surprised than I was when I kept hearing, in interview after interview, so much discussion about mental, emotional, and spiritual healing factors.

This chapter is about the emotions we hold on to from our past and their connection to our physical health. To explore this subject fully, we will first look at why suppressed emotions, particularly stress and fear, are bad for our health. From there, we will discuss the optimal way to process emotions, followed by the healing story of one Radical Remission survivor who released suppressed emotions in order to help heal his lung cancer. Finally, you will find a list of simple action steps at the end of this chapter that can help you get started with the process of unloading your own emotional baggage.

ILLNESS EQUALS BLOCKAGE

In addition to finding out *what* people do to heal their cancer, I also study *why* Radical Remission survivors do these things. I call these motivating principles "underlying beliefs," and one of the most common underlying beliefs that comes up over and over in my research is the belief that illness is a blockage on either the physical, emotional, or spiritual level of our beings. Survivors as well as alternative cancer healers believe that health is achieved when we have a state of unrestricted movement on all three of these levels. This concept gives us a new way to think about cancer, as well as a new way to think about treating it.

Let me give you an analogy to help you better understand how cancer forms in the body. A well-functioning body is a lot like a city, especially when it comes to a city's garbage collection system. Just as you have things that you throw out every day—for example, food that has spoiled—your cells also have things they throw out every day, such as toxins, bacteria, or old cell parts. And just as the garbage truck comes to your house each week to pick up your trash, your immune system stops by your cells each day to pick up their waste. In a city, garbage trucks take the trash to a local waste treatment center, where it is sorted and either recycled or discarded. Similarly, waste from your cells is taken by your immune system to organs, such as your kidney and liver, where it is then either recycled or expelled from your body.

Just as there would be serious problems if the garbage trucks in your city did not collect trash for weeks on end, serious problems arise in your body when things build up and are not processed through your waste disposal system—and that appears to be what happens with cancer. We all have cancer cells in our bodies every day; they are simply "bad copies" of cells, and that copying process can go wrong for a variety of reasons. Regardless of the reason, your immune system usually notices these bad copies and promptly removes them from your body, without any problem or cause for alarm.

Sometimes, though, either because your immune system is weakened or because cancer cells are especially good at hiding behind chemical "masks," cancer cells may not always get removed from your body as they should. When this happens over an extended period of time, the cancer cells eventually build up enough to form a tumor. From the point of view of the people I research, not only does this "blockage" of a tumor need to be removed, but also the *cause* of the blockage needs to be addressed, so things do not build up again.

Due to this belief, the Radical Remission survivors I study are very focused on clearing out anything that is "stuck" in their being, whether on the physical level, the emotional level, or the spiritual level. In their opinion, one person may have more of a physical blockage, while another person may have more of an emotional or spiritual blockage. Regardless of which level the blockage is on, however, the overarching goal is still the same: identify the blockage, figure out where it came from, and release it fully.

One of the survivors I studied who believed that his cancer was caused by a blockage on the emotional level was a man named "Adam." Adam was diagnosed with a grade 3 oligodendroglioma, an advanced type of brain tumor that has a median survival rate of only three and a half years.[1] After two grueling surgeries that removed most of his infiltrating brain tumor, Adam turned down the recommended chemotherapy and radiation because they provided such slim chances for survival and came with terrible side effects. His doctors warned him that, by refusing their advice, his cancer would likely be back within a year. Nevertheless, he decided to try other healing methods instead. So, in addition to changing his diet and taking many supplements to help clear out any physical blockages in his body, he focused on releasing emotional blockages from his past:

> *When you watch the mind pattern, or watch the thought form that created the disease to begin with, if you can find out what that is and fix* that, *then there's no way for the physical aspect of the disease to exist. . . . Wherever the cancer is, it represents a kind of resentment you're holding. . . . So, I did what I call "release work." Imagine . . . your father. You can probably think about all the things that your dad has done for you, both positive and negative. . . . But the reality is that, at a certain point, you have to release that stuff. . . . If you release that moment up into the experience of whatever this universe is, it no longer has to exist. And it doesn't have to exist inside of you anymore either. So, I did a lot of release work.*

Today, more than four years after his doctors told him his cancer would recur within a year, Adam is enjoying a cancer-free life and a satisfying career as a professional musician. To this day, he believes the most important piece of his healing was releasing the emotional blockage of resentment that was stuck in the emotional level of his body-mind-spirit system.

WHAT ARE SUPPRESSED EMOTIONS?

Suppressed emotions are *any* emotions you are hanging on to from your past, whether positive, negative, conscious, or unconscious. The most common emotions we hold on to are negative ones, such as stress, fear, trauma, regret, anger, or sadness, but we may also hold on to positive emotions, such as happiness. Most people would assume that holding on to happiness is a good thing; however, when happiness is tied to your past, it quickly turns into nostalgia, which keeps us focused on a memory of past happiness, as opposed to the possibility of actual happiness in the present.

In addition to being positive or negative, suppressed emotions may be conscious or unconscious, meaning you may not be able to remember them fully or at all. That's because traumatic memories, such as accidents or incidents of physical or sexual abuse, are often blocked from one's conscious memory. You will find suggestions for how to release such unconscious, buried memories in the "Action Steps" section at the end of this chapter, but for now, it is important to note that any emotion you are holding on to from your past is a suppressed emotion that may, over time, lead to an unhealthy blockage in your body-mind-spirit system.

"Emily" is a Radical Remission survivor who focused on releasing emotions from her past in order to help heal her cancer. She was diagnosed with stage 4 cervical cancer and agreed to have surgery, but when her doctor insisted on following up with chemotherapy and radiation in order to treat her metastases, she hesitated. Her intuition told her that her already-weak body would not be able to handle such intense treatments, and more important, her training in energy medicine led her to believe that suppressed emotions from her recent divorce might be keeping her immune system from working as well as it could:

> *I asked my doctor to give me a couple of weeks to solve this problem. I explained to him about my brutal, unexpected divorce and how, energetically speaking, that is the second chakra [an energy center, in yoga theory, located near the cervix]. Therefore, as an*

energy medicine therapist, I had a few tools that I was able to apply. My doctor gave me the opportunity to do that but told me to come back after those two weeks and have a CAT scan and other tests to be sure the cancer was gone. So, I agreed. For a couple of weeks I did Reiki, yoga, Healing Touch, prayed, cried, laughed, forgave, and—one day at a time—started clearing and dealing with grief using different energy medicine modalities. The process was truly healing on many levels.

When Emily went back for a follow-up scan just two weeks later, her doctor was shocked to see that her metastases were gone and she had no detectable cancer left in her body. Six years later (and counting), Emily is feeling happier and healthier than ever, especially now that she has released the grief of her divorce.

STRESS AND CANCER

In the last twenty years or so, research has begun to support the theory that letting go of suppressed emotions can be beneficial to the physical body. This is especially true of stress, because so many studies have focused on how that particular emotional state affects the body. One of the landmark stress studies was published in the *New England Journal of Medicine* in 1991.[2] In this study, 420 men and women first took surveys on a variety of factors, including their stress levels. Then, some of the subjects were given a nasal spray that contained saline, while the rest were given a nasal spray that contained the common cold virus (don't worry, they were all told ahead of time that this would be happening, although they did not know which spray they would get). Can you guess what happened? The ones who reported being more stressed initially developed a full-on cold, while the ones who reported being less stressed initially were better able to fight it off. Of all the factors listed in the surveys, stress was the only one that made a significant difference in the outcome. In other words, this study showed that holding on to stress makes you more vulnerable to developing disease.

Since this groundbreaking study, hundreds of other studies have shown that stress is associated not only with the common cold but also with more serious things like heart disease, autoimmune disorders, and cancer. It is still difficult for researchers to prove whether stress by itself can cause cancer, mostly because it would be unethical to make one group of people purposefully stressed and another group purposefully relaxed and then see which developed cancer. However, what researchers know for certain is that stress weakens the immune system, and the immune system plays a key role in detecting and removing cancer cells from the body.

One of the ways that stress weakens the immune system is by changing which neuropeptides our cells release. Neuropeptides are chemicals released by certain cells in your body that then latch on to other cells in your body and create an effect. Neuropeptides that have a healthy effect on your immune system include serotonin, dopamine, and relaxin; these are released whenever you feel relaxed and happy. Neuropeptides that have a weakening effect on your immune system, especially over an extended period of time, include cortisol, epinephrine, and adrenaline; these are known as the stress hormones. What makes stress—or any emotion, for that matter—so powerful is that almost *every cell in our bodies* has the ability to both produce and receive these neuropeptides.[3] In other words, the antiquated idea that the mind and body are separate is no longer scientifically accurate; instead, the mind—in the form of emotion-driven neuropeptides—is present in every cell, which means an emotion such as stress can negatively affect every cell in your body, not just your immune cells.

One of the healers I met during my research trip studies precisely this topic: how stress and the overall suppression of emotions can negatively affect any cell. Just like the Nobel laureate Otto Warburg, who we learned about in chapter 1, Dr. Tsuneo Kobayashi, an integrative oncologist in Tokyo, also believes that cancer cells are merely healthy cells whose mitochondria have become damaged. What makes him different from Dr. Warburg is that Dr. Kobayashi believes suppressing emotions is one of the key things that can damage the mitochondria.

As we learned in chapter 1, mitochondria are in charge of converting the oxygen we breathe into the energy our cells need. They are also in charge of telling our cells when it is time to die and be replaced by new cells; this is known as "programmed cell death" or "apoptosis." When someone has cancer, two things are happening: the cancerous cells are no longer getting their energy from oxygen but instead from sugar (i.e., glucose), and they are no longer dying when they should but instead replicating and living forever. Both of these functions—creating energy via oxygen and dying on time—are jobs of the mitochondria. Therefore, Dr. Warburg's and Dr. Kobayashi's theory that cancer cells are simply healthy cells whose mitochondria have been damaged makes a lot of sense—and, in fact, many other researchers today agree with them.[4]

Taking this idea even further, though, Dr. Kobayashi hypothesizes that a wide variety of things can damage a cell's mitochondria, even suppressing one's emotions:

> [Cancer] is not made by cancer cells but by human beings . . . with their bad circulation and low [core body] temperature. . . . My understanding is that cancer cells are not malignant cells but sacrificed or delinquent cells . . . adapted to the wrong circumstances. . . . In our body, cancer cells never arise in the heart or

small intestine, because the heart and small intestine are warm, with high blood circulation and high oxygen content. . . . Cancer is the end result of alexithymia—or not expressing feelings or emotions. Most cancer patients, before suffering from cancer, are suffering from alexithymia. Alexithymia [causes] blood pressure to go down and [core body] temperature to lower . . . and this destroys the functioning of the mitochondria.

Because Dr. Kobayashi sees mitochondrial damage as the main cause of cancer, his treatments therefore focus on trying to repair mitochondria. He attempts to do this in a variety of ways, using both physical treatments—such as raising one's core body temperature—and emotional treatments—such as having his patients do emotional release work.

If you are feeling stressed by what you just read about stress, I have some good news: stress management works. Studies have shown that releasing feelings of stress, anger, or fear can strengthen your immune system—and quite quickly, at that. For example, in one such study, breast cancer patients who took a ten-week stress management course showed increased white blood cell counts afterward, as compared to a control group of breast cancer patients who did not take the course.[5] In a similar study, melanoma cancer patients who participated in a six-week course that taught both stress management and relaxation techniques showed a significant increase in natural killer (NK) cell activity, as compared to a control group of melanoma patients who did not take the course.[6] This finding is especially important because NK cells are our immune systems' natural cancer cell killers. This special type of white blood cell has the ability to bind to a cancer cell and inject it with a kind of "poison" (perforin) that causes the cancer cell to die.

In addition to stress management courses, there are other ways you can reduce your stress and release suppressed emotions, and these will be listed later in this chapter. In the meantime, though, it is important to remember this: holding on to stress weakens your body's immune system and its ability to fight cancer, while releasing stress strengthens it.

FEAR AND CANCER

Among all the suppressed emotions Radical Remission survivors talk to me about releasing, fear is by far one of the most common discussed. Perhaps this is because fear is something we all have felt to some degree, whereas not everyone can relate to, for example, intensely held grief or resentment. The fear of death, in particular, is something we all must face at some point in our lives, and cancer patients are forced to face it the moment they hear the words "You have cancer."

Because fear is such a dominant emotion for most cancer patients, many of the healers I study believe it is the first thing that needs to be addressed. One of those healers is Patti Conklin, Ph.D. Patti is a "medical intuitive," which means that she apparently has the clairvoyant ability to know where, how, and why a person is sick simply by looking at that person and reading his or her energy field. She explained to me that she was born with a different kind of eyesight from most people, with the ability to view people's energy fields as one would view a TV screen of static. During our interview, I asked Patti what she thinks a cancer patient should do to begin the healing process, and she replied:

Surrender. The goal is to get the physical body, the emotional body, and the spiritual body back into alignment, back into balance. There's love and fear. And people look at fear as False

Evidence Appearing Real. I look at it as Forgetting Every Available Resource. And that resource is what we have inside of us. I encourage my patients to surrender, to be at peace with dying and be at peace with living. And the more that you can bring the body into neutrality, the greater chance you'll have of healing. . . . But if people are in fear, then the whole energy field, the subtle energy fields, the immune system—it all shuts down.

In other words, Dr. Conklin believes that releasing fear and sinking into that inherently available "resource" of internal peace can help bring the body back into balance, whereas holding on to fear can cause the body's systems to shut down, thereby creating an energetic blockage that can eventually lead to physical disease. However, truly surrendering in the way Dr. Conklin advises involves looking at one's fear of death head-on, and that is not always an easy thing to do.

For instance, "Nathan" was forced to face his own fear of death when he decided to stop chemotherapy and instead pursue alternative medicine treatments. He was originally diagnosed with stage 4 lymphoplasmacytic lymphoma, an incredibly rare and hard-to-treat form of lymphoma. Conventional medical doctors know very little about this type of cancer, so when a few rounds of chemotherapy made Nathan's cancer grow dramatically, he decided to stop. He parted ways with his conventional doctors shortly thereafter, and they regretfully informed him that he had only one to two years to live. Since then, Nathan has embarked on a healing journey that has included energy treatments from various healers, mistletoe herbal supplements, and a commitment to release all trauma from his past and all fear from his present. He describes what it was like to face his fear of death:

When I decided that I would stop [the chemotherapy], the fear really hit me hard—worse than before, because I really knew that this decision involved that I might die in the next year. . . . And there were about four days when I didn't sleep. I couldn't sleep at night when I went through this process of facing this fear and accepting that I was going to die. But after that, it was gone! The fear of death was gone. And once you make those decisions, once you jump into trust, things just happen, you know? Two days later, I just "happened" to meet [a famous healer].

Nathan's doctors gave him one to two years to live back in 2005. When I interviewed him in 2011, he was fully enjoying traveling in South America, soaking up all its natural beauty. I fully realize that facing one's fear of death can range from being quite easy to tremendously difficult, depending on your beliefs about what happens after you die. However, almost all the Radical Remission survivors I study say that facing that fear directly—at least for a short while—gave them some degree of relief, because they were no longer ignoring the elephant in the room.

To give you an example of how much power fear has over the physical body, consider this study, in which the researchers were not intending to study fear at all. Instead, they were trying figure out whether or not a new type of chemotherapy worked. They separated cancer patients into two randomized groups: the first group received the new chemotherapy, while a second, control group *thought* they were getting the new chemotherapy but were only getting saline infusions. Amazingly, 30 percent—forty people—in the control group lost all their hair, simply because they thought they were receiving chemotherapy.[7] In other words, their intense fear of having a side effect caused their bodies to produce the side effect, even though they weren't actually getting any chemotherapy.

In countless other studies researchers have shown that fear keeps the body stuck in fight-or-flight mode, which means the body cannot switch over to rest-and-repair mode. Many people don't realize that these two modes of operating are mutually exclusive; so, if you are feeling fear, your body is not healing, and if your body is self-healing, you are not feeling fear. For example, in one study people who tended to be fearful to begin with did not produce any natural killer cells after being exposed to a stressor, while people who were by nature not as fearful did produce them.[8] That is why so many radical survivors repeatedly tell me that releasing fear from the body is one of the absolute best things you can do to help your body heal, because fear literally shuts down the immune system.

THE WATERFALL SOLUTION

We will talk specifically at the end of this chapter about ways in which you can start to release suppressed emotions from your body-mind-spirit system, but the end goal is to be like a waterfall, where emotions well up in response to your present moment and then wash right through you like the water of a waterfall. In this way, you never accumulate any emotional baggage from your past, and you are able to experience each new moment from a neutral place.

Michael Broffman, a well-known licensed acupuncturist and herbalist in the San Francisco area who has treated thousands of cancer patients over the past twenty years, describes this waterfall technique:

> *We're mostly seeing Radical Remission when you can release somebody from fear. . . . The people who experience Radical Remission, and those who have been the most successful in long-term remission even if they've been called back for treatment, are those*

who have the best way of dealing with uncertainty. Uncertainty seems to be a very key aspect—people who can stay in the present and not project fear into the future [do better]. So, if you can deal with uncertainty about the cancer by staying in the present, then that seems to be the ticket. From a remission standpoint, it seems to then cause the body to relax. The body relaxes, gets more oxygen, more oxygen means the cell has a better chance, and then you'll fall in line.

In other words, Michael believes that letting go of suppressed emotions, like uncertainty and fear, and then staying peacefully centered in the present moment allows the body to relax in such a way that it actually increases the body's ability to heal.

NOW THAT WE have explored the basic concepts of releasing suppressed emotions, we will explore this topic in depth through the healing story of Joe, a man who released the emotions of his past in order to address the lung cancer of his present. As with the other healing stories featured in this book, you may find yourself challenged by some of Joe's choices, whether medical or personal. Nevertheless, I invite you to read his story with an open mind and with an eye for the larger themes.

—⟋ Joe's Story ⟍—

Joe was born into a Catholic family, lived in a Catholic neighborhood, and attended an all-boys Catholic school. Forty years later, Joe reflects on what it was like growing up like this in his typically comedic tone:

Twelve years of Catholic school taught me a lot about God. First,
he was most definitely a he. *He was white, perhaps northern*
European. He was very old and had a white beard. He was
judgmental and could get very angry. And his punishments were
much more severe than anything my parents or the sisters at my
school could dole out. [laughs]

Of course, not all Catholics feel this way, but for Joe, that was his
experience. As a child, he was taught to fear a God who would love
you as long as you did not sin, but who would send you to eternal hell
if you did something wrong. In Joe's words, "God scared the crap out
of me." And Joe felt like this even before he realized he was gay.

As you might imagine, adolescence was a troubling time for Joe.
He tried to suppress his feelings for other boys and was so ashamed
that he could not even bring himself to confess his thoughts to the
priest. Joe told no one of his "terrible" secret and prayed desperately
for God to remove the sinful thoughts from his head. Despite his
earnest efforts, his prayers went unanswered. He tried his best to
rein in his feelings, but as early adolescence turned into late adolescence, he occasionally gave in to his feelings and became physically
intimate with another gay teen. Afterward, he felt intense shame
and fear and swore he would never sin again.

Given this situation, it is perhaps not surprising that Joe turned
to drugs and alcohol to escape his belief that God hated him. He
began smoking cigarettes, which quickly became a habit, and he
even considered suicide at one point—until he remembered that
hell was the punishment for that, too. The only solution he could
think of was to leave the Catholic Church somehow. So, when
choosing colleges, he purposely chose a public university that had
a coed population of diverse nationalities and religions, thinking
that he might feel better about himself if he were not constantly

reminded of his sinful nature. Despite this well-thought-out plan, though, his feelings of guilt and shame ran too deeply, and they relentlessly followed him to college:

> *Even though I was in this different world [of college], I still did not feel safe to be myself, to love myself. I couldn't escape God. He was watching my every move. I went through multiple one-night stands for several years. I was afraid to get too close to another man, or this thing would take over and I would never be "normal."*

On one of his summer breaks, Joe worked as a counselor at a camp for kids with behavioral problems. He found deep meaning and fulfillment helping troubled children, and—as an added perk—he felt that God might actually approve of this new vocational calling. He remembers thinking, *Maybe service to others will look good on my "spiritual resume." Maybe on Judgment Day, God will overlook that other thing.* Feeling like he was on the right track at last, he had sex with a woman for the first time that summer. However, it took him only one time to know with certainty that he was indeed gay. In order to reconcile this realization, he decided to abandon his religion completely. He recalls that period of time:

> *It took several more years, but I eventually fell in love with a man for the first time. There was no turning back. I couldn't continue to deny myself the experience of a loving relationship. In order for me to be happy, I had to leave God out of the equation.*

After college, Joe abandoned Catholicism and moved to a gay-friendly city, launched a career helping others, and began a long-term relationship with a man. Over the years, although he gradually stopped believing in hell, he still envied his friends who spoke of a deep spiritual connection with the divine. As the years passed, his long-term relationship eventually became rocky and his job often left him feeling burned out. By the time he was in his forties, he was no longer in a positive mental space and had come to view life as "something to be endured."

———————

THIS WAS THE state of things in March of 2007, when Joe was preparing for one of the few true joys in his life: travel. He was about to go on a much-anticipated vacation to Peru and needed some vaccinations before he left. He had recently quit smoking in an effort to get healthier, but his doctor still smelled smoke on his breath and therefore recommended a CT scan to get a baseline reading of Joe's lungs. The results were devastating. There were a dozen spots on each lung and two enlarged lymph nodes, indicating the very worst: metastatic lung cancer.

Joe went to Peru thinking this could possibly be his last trip, and then he underwent several months of testing. In June, the doctors finally performed a minor surgery to biopsy one of his tumors. This confirmed his diagnosis as metastatic, non-small-cell lung cancer. His doctors recommended three rounds of chemotherapy using a cocktail of multiple drugs, followed by a surgery that would involve cracking his ribs open and removing a dozen lymph nodes, then six weeks of radiation to his chest. The surgeon told him this was an aggressive form of cancer that therefore needed to be treated aggressively.

Before beginning such intense medical treatment, Joe asked about his odds. His doctor told him that, even with all the treatment, 25 percent of people with his diagnosis still died within a year, 50 percent died within two years, and 80 percent died within five years. If Joe chose no treatment, he would most likely die in one to two years. He describes the morbid thoughts that went through his head at this moment:

> *I wasn't afraid of death anymore, because my view of God had matured. I no longer believed in a place called hell . . . but I had always viewed life as an experience to be endured. So, maybe this was my escape? No more problems, no more stress—finally I could feel peace.*

Joe needed some time to think, so he asked his doctors if he could take one last, brief trip. His friends happened to be going to Thailand, and they had invited him to go along. Knowing the chemotherapy, surgery, and radiation would not allow him to travel for months or possibly years, he jumped at this final chance to travel. His doctors granted his request, as long as he agreed to start chemo as soon as he returned from his trip, to which he agreed wholeheartedly.

———

WITH HEAVY THOUGHTS of the impending cancer treatment on his mind, Joe set off on what he assumed would be his last trip abroad. He was the type of person who saved up his money and vacation days carefully in order to take fun trips to new countries. This trip was somewhat enjoyable, although it was understandably difficult for him to relax fully and be happy. Toward the end of the trip, he spent a few days in Bangkok. While there, he was walking down a busy street when someone unexpectedly called out to him:

> *"Sir! Sir, I must speak to you!" I just kept walking, because somebody's always trying to sell you something. He followed me*

for about two blocks and finally caught up to me at the light. I turned around and it was this Sikh guy, with a black turban and a black beard. He said, "Sir, as you walked past, God told me that I had to tell you your fortune." . . . I was very *skeptical. I don't believe in that kind of stuff. But then he looked me straight in the eyes and said, "Although you look very healthy, the doctors have told you that you're very sick and that you might die. But don't believe them, because I see that you're going to live until you're eighty-eight, and then you'll die suddenly."*

Regardless of Joe's skepticism, the man's accurate comment about his health status made Joe pause. Out of curiosity more than anything, he agreed to sit with this fortune-teller for a reading. The man then proceeded to baffle him with insanely accurate descriptions of his various relationships, familial, friendly, and romantic. He went on to describe his current long-term relationship with stunning accuracy, explaining the hardships that he and his partner had endured and continued to struggle with. Joe explains his reaction:

By this point, he was freaking me out. He ended by telling me that I would meet a red-haired woman who would lead me to health. I emptied my pocket of the last of my [Thai] money and returned to my hotel with my mind racing. I had a terrible time sleeping that night. All of my previously held beliefs were shaken.

On his first day back at work, Joe told a coworker about his experience with the strange fortune-teller. The coworker immediately reached up to her bulletin board, took down a business card, and handed it to Joe. She said it was the card of a local energy healer who came highly recommended, although she herself had never been to see her. Joe immediately e-mailed the woman, told her the fortune-teller story, and asked, "Are you my redhead?" She replied, "Yes, I am!" So, on a whim, Joe made an appointment for the following week, while his chemo was scheduled to start in ten days.

Joe found this healer to be a young, energetic woman with reddish-brown hair and magenta highlights. *Close enough,* he jokingly thought to himself. After he told her about his advanced lung cancer, she recommended an energy treatment to help clear his chakras and realign his energy. She spent the next hour gently shaking his arms, legs, and torso, while also talking to him about his health condition. Joe describes:

> As she was working on me, she asked if I believed in reincarnation. I said I thought it was a possibility. She told me that my partner and I have had several incarnations together, and that in this life we made a pact to suffer together. When you look at our [rocky] history, this made sense. She explained that everything is made up of vibrational energy, and that lung cancer is often a result of unresolved anger and resentment.

At the end of the treatment, Joe was still skeptical, but he did feel much less anxious than he had when he arrived, so he decided to make another appointment to see her the next week. In the meantime, he read a book about death and dying that she had recommended called *Home with God* by Neale Donald Walsch. He found the book so engaging that he finished it in three days. Joe explains:

> [The book] painted a picture of God which made much more sense to me: a God of immeasurable love rather than the angry and vengeful God of my upbringing. I now think that man has created God in the image of himself, rather than vice versa.

The next week Joe went to start his chemotherapy. However, his oncologist first requested that he get another CT scan, so they could have a more accurate baseline. To everyone's complete surprise, the scan showed a slight shrinkage of the tumors as compared to the scan that had been taken just before Joe's trip to Thailand. Shocked but encouraged, Joe dared to ask his oncologist:

"Can we wait six months?" And [the doctor] said, "I wouldn't recommend it, because you have a very aggressive form of cancer." And the surgeon who did the biopsy told me that I was a fool [to postpone treatment], that I'd be dead in a year if I didn't get treatment.

Despite their warnings, the slight shrinking of the tumors gave Joe enough courage to postpone the chemotherapy while he continued his energy treatments with the local healer. During the next six months, he also tried any other treatments his friends suggested. For example, a woman he knew was offering Reiki energy treatments, so he began getting Reiki on a weekly basis, which he enjoyed very much. Another friend told him that high doses of vitamin C helps inhibit cancer cell growth, so he began taking that, and he started drinking kombucha tea because he had heard it was good for cancer.

He also saw a different holistic healer a few times, one recommended by a close friend. This healer, like the first one, had an uncanny ability to tell him things about his life and his relationships with incredible accuracy. A recurring theme in what both of these healers said to him was that unprocessed, suppressed emotions could contribute to physical illness. When Joe also read in a spiritual book that lung cancer could be associated with unresolved anger and resentment, it got him thinking. Why had his long-term relationship been so rocky? And did the guilt he felt toward the Catholic God of his childhood have anything to do with his cancer? The idea that his smoking caused his cancer was obvious to him, but these ideas about emotions were new to him, and much more subtle.

So, Joe spent the remainder of the six months focused not only on realigning the energy of his chakras and taking vitamin C and other supplements, but also on letting go of any anger or resentment he felt toward his partner or toward God. When the six months were up and it was time for his next CT scan, he was hopeful that it would show even more shrinkage of his tumors, but he honestly wasn't sure what to expect. The results came back and, to his delight, they showed more slight shrinkage of his tumors. He was relieved and excited by these positive results, and once again asked if he could postpone chemotherapy. Baffled as they were, his doctors simply shook their heads in wonder and agreed to let him continue with "whatever he was doing."

SO, OVER THE next six months, Joe continued on with his energy treatments and supplements, but he also read more spiritual books in an attempt to start releasing the deep-seated shame, sadness, and anger he had felt toward God ever since his Catholic upbringing. In contrast, these new spiritual books described a nonjudgmental God and talked about connecting to the divinity inside oneself. The six months passed quickly, and soon it was time for another CT scan. This scan again showed even more shrinkage of his tumors, so he asked for another six months to continue his journey of healing and spiritual redefining.

This time, Joe moved on from spiritual books and started experimenting with spiritual practices, such as meditation, in order to try to release the entrenched emotions of his past. During this time, he decided to attend a ten-day silent meditation retreat at a nearby Buddhist center. Rumor had it that this ten-day course, replete with 4:30 A.M. wake-up calls and fourteen hours of meditation per day, was a "fast track to enlightenment." Enlightenment sounded great to Joe, so he signed up for the retreat even though he had always had difficulty meditating. As he describes, "My previous attempts at meditation were always short periods of trying not to think followed by long periods thinking about how hard it is not to think."

At the meditation retreat, the attendees were told to sit in silence, close their eyes, and focus their attention on their nostrils, all the while noticing any sensations that came up and trying not to react to those sensations. Every time they caught their minds wandering, they were told to focus again on their nostrils. As is to be expected, this was very difficult for Joe:

The first day was hard. *I had never sat on a pillow on the floor for twelve hours in one day before. The second day was even worse. I began to feel anger flowing up from every ounce of my being. It took all of the strength I had to keep from running out to my car and back to my reality. Reality was much more tolerable than this. The teacher kept preparing us for the third day, when the true vipassana meditation would begin. I convinced myself that I could make it to the third day. The rage inside me continued to boil. I had no idea where it was coming from.*

On the third day, they were instructed to silently scan their bodies from head to toe, but Joe was unable to do this because there was so much inexplicable anger still raging inside him. On the fourth day, they were led through three hour-long meditations during which they were not supposed to move at all, even if they had an itch or felt like shifting into a different position. This was also difficult for Joe. After only five minutes, he reluctantly scratched an intense itch on his back. Day five was not much better. This time he lasted only ten minutes before scratching an itch. On day six, he finally saw some progress. The inexplicable anger dissipated and he succeeded in not moving a muscle for one entire hour. Encouraged, he finally felt ready to try adding in the silent body scan. So, after the next break, he sat down, found a comfortable position, and began mentally scanning his body. After about ten minutes of this slow scanning, he suddenly began to feel something entirely different and wonderful:

I began to feel a slight tingling in my body. Suddenly, I saw a flash of light in my eyelids. In this light, I could see what I can only describe as rivers of energy. Simultaneously with what I was seeing, I was also feeling the rivers of energy throughout my entire body. What was previously aching or itching was now throbbing with pulses of pure pleasure. It lasted about three seconds. As I began to move, it returned for about another ten seconds before I came back to my "real" sensations of aches, pains, and itches. What just happened?! I thought. That was the most incredible sensation I had ever experienced! It was so beautiful and pleasurable. I had to get it back! For the rest of the hour, I scanned furiously without success. I went to bed that night with an overwhelming feeling of peace and joy. Was I hallucinating? Did I experience God? Whatever it was, I wanted more.

Eager to understand more about his "rivers of energy" experience, Joe signed up for an individual meeting with the meditation teacher the next day. He told the teacher about his blissful experience and how frustrated he was that he could not get it back. The teacher smiled and explained that many people meditate for years and never have that experience.

> *I asked him, "Did I experience God?" He smiled and said, "Some*
> *people may call it God." He continued, explaining that I had*
> *experienced my essential being below the level of my mind. The*
> *Buddha taught that we are not our bodies and we are also not*
> *our minds. "Be the observer of your mind," [said the Buddha].*

The teacher went on to explain to Joe that when the mind labels something as "good," it starts to crave it. In response, the deeper being creates experiences that involve craving. When the mind labels something as "bad," it tries to avoid it. In response, the deeper being creates experiences that involve avoiding. Therefore, because Joe's mind had labeled the blissful meditation experience as "good," it then started to crave it, and his deeper being responded by giving him an experience of just that: craving that blissful experience. The teacher ended his explanation with a suggestion not to judge or label any experiences but simply to experience them and move on. Despite this wise advice, it was very hard for Joe not to want to have that feeling again. As he puts it, "How can you possibly not crave God?" He now describes the retreat as the most difficult and life-changing event he has ever experienced:

> *I now realize that all of the anger and rage I was experiencing*
> *[at the retreat] was my anger toward God. . . . As far back as*
> *I can remember, I have viewed life as an experience to endure.*
> *Although I had experienced many joys and appreciated the*
> *positive aspects of life, my focus had always been on the half-*
> *empty glass. By focusing on the negative, I discounted the positive.*
> *I believe now that this attitude was formed at a young age, when*

*I was taught that I am separate from God. I now realize that
if God is the alpha and the omega, then that must include me.
It's impossible for me to be separate from God except in my own
mind.*

The retreat helped Joe fully release his feelings of sadness, shame,
and anger, which he realized had been brewing ever since he felt
rejected by God in his early childhood. In addition, he believes that
he felt the divine energy inside all of us when he experienced those
rivers of energy for ten seconds during the retreat. Finally, the Buddhist teacher's guidance led him to believe that thoughts and emotions can play a powerful role in determining whether life's events
are labeled as "enjoyable" or "not enjoyable":

*I now believe that God has given us free will to create our lives
and our world as we wish. . . . If you focus on the negative, that's
what you will see, despite positive things happening all around
you. If you focus on the positive, the positive will predominate,
even though the usual negative happenings in life will still
occur. . . . I've come to realize that I have control over everything
that happens in my life, and it's basically through my attitude
and my thoughts. We create everything. There is no real solid
stuff—it's all energy that's vibrating into a solid. And it's your
thoughts that create everything. So, we're God's reality show!
[laughs]*

In other words, Joe believes that thoughts are a vibration of
energy, and that vibration affects everything around it, even physical cells. For example, when I asked him what he believed was the
primary cause of his healing, he responded immediately, "My
change in attitude." And when I asked about what may have caused
his cancer, he replied without hesitation:

I created it through my thoughts, through my negativity about life in general. I felt that my life was hopeless. . . . I believe my mind has kept me blind to the presence of God all around and within me. . . . I now see life as an experience to experience, and my cup runneth over. I am learning to let go of the past and appreciate the experiences that have brought me to the present moment. I no longer feel separate from God. I see God wherever I look. I see God in the face of everyone I meet. I see God in the mirror.

Since the life-changing meditation retreat, Joe has been focusing on letting go of every ounce of anger and pessimism from his past and embracing the positive aspect of whatever he encounters in the present moment, all while still enjoying weekly Reiki sessions and traveling whenever he has accumulated enough vacation days. He still gets a CT scan every six months, and so far, they have all shown that his tumors have either shrunk slightly or held steady. While his tumors have not gone away completely, they have caused him no problems since his diagnosis, which was now over five years ago.

Joe's oncologist admits that he's completely stunned as to why Joe's aggressive form of cancer is not behaving as it "should," and he has encouraged Joe to keep doing "whatever he's doing." Meanwhile, the surgeon who told Joe he would die in a year if he did not get conventional medical treatment simply shakes her head in bafflement whenever she sees him at the hospital for his biannual CT scans. Joe describes his new way of living life in these six-month increments:

I think that I am eventually going to die of cancer, but I've decided that I'm not ready yet. So, every time I get a CT scan and it's clear, I plan another trip. That's what kind of keeps me

going. I think [that] when I run out of places I want to see, then
maybe things will change. You know? [laughs]

When Joe said this at the end of our interview, I jokingly told
him that perhaps he would die of cancer as he predicts—but not
until he is eighty-eight.

————

TO THIS DAY, Joe is one of the funniest, lighthearted people I have
ever met. That is why it is hard for me to imagine him as the
pessimistic, burned-out person he says he was before his cancer
diagnosis. Regardless of one's views on religion, smoking, or homo-
sexuality, the big picture remains that a person with advanced lung
cancer found a way to heal without conventional medicine—and
that is a case worth investigating.

Action Steps

Releasing emotions that are suppressed in the body-mind-spirit
system is no easy task, especially because we are not always aware
of which emotions we are holding on to, or from where they came.
Nevertheless, if this chapter has inspired you to clear out the emotional baggage from your past in order to boost your immune
system and increase your happiness, here are some suggestions to
get you started:

- *Keep a thought journal.* This is a popular homework activity in cognitive-behavioral therapy (CBT), which is a type
  of psychotherapy that asks you to take a closer look at your
  underlying thoughts and their subsequent emotional reactions. To start a thought journal, take some time at lunch and
  at bedtime for two straight weeks to write down all the emo-

tional events of your day, both positive and negative. Then try to write down what you were thinking *just before* you felt that emotion.

The idea in CBT is that our underlying thoughts cause us to feel happy or sad, yet many of us are not aware of what our underlying thoughts are. For example, people who suffer from depression are often surprised when they keep a thought journal to find out that their most common, underlying thoughts are *I'm a failure at everything I do* or *The world is an inherently dangerous place.* At this point, finding a good CBT therapist to work with, or at least using a CBT workbook, can help you release underlying beliefs that no longer serve you.

- *Make a list of your emotional moments.* Take some time one evening to write down all the most emotional moments from your past, as far back as you can remember, both positive and negative. When you are finished, look over the list and re-member the events as fully as you are able to (warning: tissues may be necessary). Then, when you are ready, have your own fire-burning ceremony and burn the list; in doing so, mentally release any suppressed emotions left over from those events.

- *Practice daily forgiveness.* When you wake up each morning, think of someone from your past or present to forgive, even if it is for something minor. If it helps, you can write down the person's name each day. If you can't think of anyone to forgive, simply forgive yourself for any wrongs you might have done before this present moment.

- *Take a stress management course.* Enroll in either a local or online stress management course for four to eight weeks in order to focus on this important life skill. One popular course is called Mindfulness-Based Stress Reduction (MBSR), which incorporates meditation into traditional stress management techniques.

- *See a healer or therapist.* If available in your local area, find a qualified energy healer or psychotherapist you can see for at least a brief time, with the goal of purposefully releasing any suppressed emotions from your past. Specific energy healing modalities that specialize in this include energy kinesiology and the BodyTalk system.

- *Try hypnosis or EMDR.* In order to release emotions from your body that you cannot consciously remember (e.g., from a childhood accident or trauma), it may be necessary to use modalities such as hypnosis or EMDR (a form of hypnosis that stands for eye movement desensitization and reprocessing). You may have to drive to your nearest city in order to find a qualified practitioner, but it will be well worth it if you can release an emotional memory you are not consciously aware of but is nonetheless affecting your physical health.

———————

THE MAIN MESSAGE I want you to take away from this chapter is not that we should never feel fear, anger, grief, stress, etc., but rather that we should try not to hold on to any particular emotion—be it positive or negative—for too long. Emotions should flow through the body like waves crashing on a beach—in and then out. We are all bound to feel sad, fearful, or angry at various points in our lives, and often these emotions are very appropriate given the situation. What Joe and the other survivors and healers I study tell me is that we shouldn't bury these feelings inside, because doing so can have a negative impact on the physical body, especially the immune system.

Emotions are a fundamental aspect of our lives; they are an important part of what makes us human. The goal is not to force ourselves to feel 100 percent happy all the time, but rather to let all types of emotions—whether positive or negative—flow in, through, and out of us, so that nothing from the past is carried over into the present, and each moment can be an opportunity for a new emotional experience.

CHAPTER 6

INCREASING POSITIVE EMOTIONS

The purpose of our lives is to be happy.

—HIS HOLINESS THE FOURTEENTH DALAI LAMA

The secret to a good life may be as simple as one word: happiness. When we feel happy and loving, our physical bodies are flooded with cancer-fighting immune cells, our emotional lives are free of stress and worry, and our social and work relationships improve. The survivors I study work diligently to find ways of increasing the amount of love, joy, and happiness they feel in the present moment. It is important to note that releasing emotions that are held in the body, such as stress, fear, anger, regret, and sadness, is quite different from what this chapter explores. Releasing suppressed emotions from the past does not necessarily mean that you will increase the amount of positive emotions in your present, although it certainly paves the way for that to happen.

In this chapter, we will explore what positive emotions are and how they affect our immune systems. Next, we'll discuss two important aspects of increasing positive emotions before we dive into the healing story of a stage 4 cancer patient who considered daily happiness to be her most important medicine. Finally, I will give you a simple prescription for fun, based on what I have learned from the people I work with, that will help bring more joy and happiness into your daily life.

WHAT ARE POSITIVE EMOTIONS?

The positive emotions Radical Remission survivors try to experience on a daily basis are happiness, joy, and love. The definitions of the words "happiness" and "joy" most people can agree on, but the use of the word "love" in this chapter may require further explanation.

In this book, I discuss three types of love. The first type is the feeling you get when you love yourself, your life, and others. It is a feeling of love that comes from within you and that you then project outward into your life. The second type of love is received by you from others; it is also called "social support." I purposefully separated these two kinds of love—that which you *give* to yourself and others versus that which you *receive*—because the participants in my research talk about them as two distinct actions, and also because not everyone excels at both. Finally, the third type of love, discussed in chapter 8, is an unconditional and spiritual type of love, which has no sense of separateness, no sense of "you" or "I."

This chapter focuses on the first type of love, which is the love, along with the happiness and joy, you create in your own life and then spread to others. One Radical Remission survivor who really focuses on this first type of love is Efrat Livny. Efrat was diagnosed with stage 3C ovarian cancer at the age of forty-nine, ironically only four years after she had left her high-stress job in order to enjoy life more. While she used a wide variety of both conventional and alternative treatments in order to address her cancer, increasing positive emotions was, for her, one of the most important steps she took:

From the very early stages of my cancer journey, it was clear to me that I would not declare battle but rather find ways to accept and befriend this new and unexpected chapter in my life. I knew that in order to do so, what I needed most was to find gratitude, joy, and fun in my life—as often and as much as I was able. Chemo presented a huge challenge for me. I could feel fear and resistance welling up in me as I prepared for my first treatment. Somehow, in the midst of it all, I thought that the right pair of shoes would make all the difference. So, I got myself a pair of purple Converse high-tops. They made me smile when I walked into that room. . . . It was those things—joy, fun, kindness, and gratitude—that became my true medicine.

Efrat has now been cancer-free for more than twelve years, and she still makes sure that joy, love, and happiness are part of her daily health regimen. Like Efrat, many of the alternative healers I study also talk about the importance of increasing positive emotions in order to help the body heal. One such healer is a meditation teacher and acupuncturist from China named Li Xin, who advises his cancer patients this way:

[Cancer patients] should pay attention not on the treatment but on bettering their normal life. When they change like this, then everything will change. . . . Even if they have chemo or radiation and they are very sick, they should try their best to make the time to go out and do meditation or qigong—something really life-giving.

For people like Efrat Livny and Li Xin, finding ways to increase the amount of happiness and joy you experience in your daily life is a vital part of the physical healing process.

WHAT HAPPENS TO OUR BODIES WHEN
WE FEEL POSITIVE EMOTIONS?

Researchers now know there is an immediate and powerful connection between the mind and the body. First, our deep-seated beliefs lead us to feel emotions—such as fear, stress, joy—that create instant bursts of hormones in our brains, and these hormones then tell our bodies what to do. When we feel fear or stress, our hormones tell the cells in our bodies to either fight or flee. When we feel joy or love, our hormones tell our bodies to spend time repairing broken cells, digesting food, and healing infections. As we learned in chapter 5, these two modes are mutually exclusive—our bodies are either fighting/fleeing or healing, not both. So, in order to turn on the body's healing mode, we must first turn off the fight-or-flight mode, and one powerful way to do this is to release suppressed emotions from the past.

As soon as we are out of fight-or-flight mode, the body naturally begins to repair cells and heal itself. However, we can "turn up" that healing—much like turning up the volume on a stereo—by purposefully trying to feel positive emotions, such as love, joy, and happiness. That's because positive emotions are like rocket fuel for the immune system. Whenever we feel the emotions of love, joy, or happiness, the glands in our brains release a surge of healing hormones into our bloodstreams, including serotonin, relaxin, oxytocin, dopamine, and endorphins.[1] These hormones instantly communicate with all the cells in our bodies, telling them to do things such as:

- Lower blood pressure, heart rate, and cortisol (the stress hormone)

- Improve blood circulation

- Deepen our breathing, which brings more oxygen to each cell
- Digest our food more slowly, which helps the body absorb more nutrients
- Increase white and red blood cell activity, which helps the immune system
- Increase natural killer cell activity, which helps the immune system fight cancer
- Clear out any infections
- Scan for cancer and remove any cancer cells

All these amazing physical changes have been documented in clinical studies, in which researchers do things like count people's number of immune cells before and after showing them a comedy video.[2] The reason this list is so relevant to cancer patients is that all these changes have also been shown to improve significantly the immune system's ability to remove cancer cells.[3] Laughter has even been shown to increase the number of immune cells of people undergoing chemotherapy.[4] Similar studies have shown that people who are battling an illness and have an overall positive attitude live significantly longer than people who are battling an illness and are pessimistic.[5] In other words, study after study is finding evidence to back up the old saying "Happy people live longer."

A spiritual healer I studied from Hawaii named Murali believes so firmly in the power of positive emotions to boost the immune system, she recommends that all her cancer patients send love directly to their cancer cells:

Once you're beginning to feel comfortable about non-resistance [to your cancer], your second step would be more and more of an

intended feeling of love directed visually [toward your cancer]. . . .
Your body does not know the difference between feeling good with
a smile that's genuine—let's say you're watching a comedy and just
naturally smiling—or intending one [a smile]. And when you do
that, guess what happens? Endorphins! Big, beautiful, loving endor-
phins that send all these healing messages to the cells. . . . If you
could see it physically, you would actually be looking at streams of
endorphins rushing, feel-good hormones rushing, rushing to create
much more loving energy.

When Murali suggested this during our interview, I explained to
her that many of the cancer patients I work with would be afraid
that sending love to their cancer cells would make them grow even
faster. Murali instantly responded that sending love to cancer cells
in this way would actually repair them and return them to their
natural, healthy state. Her hypothesis could very well be accurate,
since we already know that endorphins help heal damaged cells by
both decreasing inflammation and increasing the immune cell activity around damaged cells.[6]

Many of the other healers I have interviewed from around the
world agree with Murali. They believe that cancer cells are simply
healthy cells that have been damaged and need to be repaired.
Western medicine agrees that cancer cells have been damaged—
either by a toxin, virus, bacteria, or genetic mutation—but it also
believes that cancer cells are beyond repair, and therefore the only
option is to kill them. That is why almost all cancer research for the
past hundred years has looked for the best way to kill cancer cells,
whether by chemotherapy, radiation, or surgery.

Meanwhile, there has been very little research done on whether
or not damaged cancer cells can be *rehabilitated* into healthy cells.
However, at least one recent and groundbreaking study may prove

the healers right. In this study,[7] early-stage prostate cancer patients who voluntarily chose not to undergo immediate medical treatment were randomly split into two groups. The first group did "watchful waiting" for their cancer, meaning they received no medical treatment and instead were closely monitored. The second group tried an alternative regimen that included a vegetable-rich diet, daily exercise, and emotional practices designed to release stress and increase happiness. In case you were worried, both groups were closely monitored so that anyone whose cancer suddenly flared up could drop out of the study immediately and begin chemotherapy.

In the watchful-waiting group, six men had to drop out and start chemotherapy because their cancer flared up. In the alternative-treatment group, zero men had their cancer flare up; in fact, their tumor markers decreased by an average of 4 percent, whereas the watchful-waiting group's markers *increased* by 6 percent. Perhaps most impressive, though, was a follow-up study, which found that men in the alternative-treatment group who had previously had a prostate cancer gene turned *on* now had that gene turned *off*—after only three months of being on the alternative-treatment regimen.[8] In other words, these studies showed that by participating in the alternative program—which included increasing positive emotions—prostate cancer patients were able to turn off their cancer genes *and* reduce the amount of cancer already in their bodies.

While it remains unclear whether the alternative-treatment regimen helped the men's immune systems kill cancer cells or instead rehabilitate them into healthy cells, these studies—and all the studies listed in this section—show us that strengthening the immune system by doing things such as increasing positive emotions can significantly help your body fight cancer.

HAPPINESS IS A HABIT

When Radical Remission survivors talk to me about trying to feel more love, joy, and happiness in order to help their bodies heal, they talk about it as they would talk about flossing their teeth or working out: they see happiness as a habit you have to practice daily in order to reap the desired benefits. This is an important idea, because most people in our culture assume that happiness is something we're either born with or we're not, that we're stuck as either glass-half-full or glass-half-empty people. The survivors and healers I study would disagree. They believe we can *all* experience consistent joy in our lives, as long as we practice feeling happy on a daily basis.

For most of the Radical Remission survivors I study, feeling happy was a nearly impossible thing to do immediately after hearing their cancer diagnoses. However, they quickly realized that staying locked in fear day after day would neither be enjoyable nor helpful to their immune systems. So, at first they had to force themselves to do things that would turn off their fear and turn on some joy, even if only for a few minutes. For example, some of them chose to watch a funny YouTube video, go to an afternoon yoga class, or call up someone they loved. Little by little, they purposefully increased these kinds of activities until that feeling of happiness was filling up more and more minutes of each day. What they discovered is that, by purposefully making time every day to do something that brought them joy, the quicker that feeling of joy came to them and the longer its pleasant effects lasted throughout the day. In this way, doing activities that brought them joy was similar to taking pain medicine in that it made them feel noticeably better.

One survivor who regularly focused on increasing his positive emotions is "Allen." Allen was only forty when he was diagnosed with stage 2 head and neck cancer, and although he agreed to have the main tumor surgically removed from his neck, his intuition told him not to do the recommended chemo and radiation, much to his doctor's dismay. Instead, he decided to embark on an intense self-healing program, which included, among other things, focusing on his emotions:

> *I experienced profound changes in my very being. My thoughts and emotions were radically different as I experienced a total paradigm shift in my existence. . . . I cherished my children, myself, and the very moment that is "now" like never before. . . . I acquired a sense of perspective, and through intense introspection and study, I was able to achieve a paradigm shift in my consciousness. This had a cascade effect upon my entire existence—nothing was the same.*

By making time each day to appreciate the present moment, Allen began to be filled with emotions such as love and gratitude, which eventually became so strong that his entire life changed for the better. With the help of other changes (e.g., diet), it has now been five years (and counting), and Allen currently has no evidence of disease.

In a similar vein, Carlos Sauer, a shamanic healer from Brazil, describes the importance of making happiness a daily habit in this way:

> *[You take] a new look at the sunrise, or you look at the new day, and you say, "Thank you, God. Thank you, Creator, for this wonderful new day. I've never, ever seen it before. This is a brand new day! Today is going to be a great day. It's already a great day." . . . The only thing we have is today—right now—so, I try to do everything I can to enjoy every minute of my day. . . . To be*

in good health has a lot to do with happiness. Your health is connected to your happiness.

Like so many of the other healers I interview, Carlos believes a daily dose of happiness is one of the most important "medicines" you can take.

YOU DON'T HAVE TO FEEL HAPPY ALL THE TIME

Please keep in mind that making a commitment to feeling happy for at least five minutes a day is not the same thing as thinking you need to feel happy *all day, every day* in order to improve your health. This is a tragic and misguided conclusion that has sprung out of the mind-body medicine movement, such that many cancer patients feel guilty whenever they are stressed or scared, because they know that these emotions can weaken the immune system. Can you imagine the pressure of having to feel happy all of the time, especially when dealing with a life-threatening illness?

It is true that stress, fear, grief, and anger have weakening effects on the immune system. However, it never made sense to me to cover up valid feelings of fear with a false veneer of positivity along with an additional layer of guilt. That's why I was so pleased to learn that most Radical Remission survivors and alternative healers believe it is healthiest for a person to feel fully, and then *release* fully, any and all emotions that come up, whether they be positive or negative. Doing so allows you not only to experience the full range of human expression, but also to spend more time feeling truly happy in between the various waves of emotion. Young toddlers are a great example of this—they can be flooded with anger one moment, and after feeling it fully and releasing it, they will be completely happy five minutes later.

All of the Radical Remission survivors I have met experienced days, or even months, that were filled with pain, fear, or sadness. When you are facing death, it is almost impossible not to feel this way. However, even on the most difficult days, they still force themselves to try to find at least a few moments of happiness or laughter. One of the Radical Remission survivors I interviewed found a clever way of doing this. Janet Jacobsen was diagnosed at age sixty with uterine cancer. She could not have been more shocked with her diagnosis, because at that time she felt incredibly happy, ate well, and exercised regularly. After a few years of combining both complementary and conventional medicine, including surgery, chemo, and radiation, her cancer unfortunately recurred. That is when she committed fully to healing herself and dove wholeheartedly into alternative approaches. Three years later (and counting), Janet has since learned the importance of bringing humor and playfulness into her healing journey, especially when negative emotions come up:

> *Play is a powerful shift tool when I'm stuck in negative patterns. When I notice my cynical attitude taking over, I play with it. I give it a name—Cynny—and I exaggerate her grousing. I let her rip! This brings her out of the shadows, into the light, into wholeness, and I expand into the playful, prayerful state of grace. Plus, it's just plain fun.*

Janet discovered what many other Radical Remission survivors have discovered, that there is a fine line between cynicism and optimism, and only a small amount of effort is required to switch between the two.

NOW THAT WE have discussed what positive emotions are and why they are such powerful stimulants for your immune system, especially when you make them a daily habit, I would like to share with you the healing story of Saranne Rothberg. Saranne is a stage 4 breast cancer survivor who made a commitment to feel happy at least twice a day, every day, no matter how hard things got during her cancer journey. As you will see, Saranne also used all eight of the other key factors listed in this book in order to heal her cancer. However, increasing positive emotions was, at least in her opinion, the primary and guiding force behind her Radical Remission.

—⟋ Saranne's Story ⟍—

In 1993, Saranne Rothberg was twenty-nine years old and in love with her first child, a beautiful newborn girl named Lauriel. Despite this new joy, Saranne was dealing with many stressors in her life, including a strained marriage, a blind mother, an elderly father, and a grandmother who had recently fallen ill—all while Saranne was working as a television consultant. During this time, Saranne was also dealing with what her doctors believed was a recurrent breast infection caused by breastfeeding. Over the next few years, Saranne endured the death of her mother and grandmother, as well as an emotionally painful divorce, all of which gave her very little time to focus on the "breast infection" that was making her feel worse every day.

In 1999, after having seen eleven different doctors in six years, Saranne was finally given the correct diagnosis: it was a malignant breast tumor, not a breast infection. At first, her doctors told her it was likely stage 2 breast cancer, and there was no apparent lymph node involvement. However, further testing soon revealed the worst possible scenario: it was actually stage 4 breast cancer, and it had not only spread to her lymph nodes but also formed small metastases above and under her aorta and possibly on her neck and spine.

When Saranne heard this news, she was absolutely terrified. Her doctor told her on a Friday afternoon, but she was not able to meet with her new oncologist until Monday. Knowing she would be facing this grave diagnosis all alone, with only her five-year-old daughter by her side, Saranne felt overwhelmed in the face of the oncoming ordeal. Then, suddenly, she remembered something:

> *I knew about the life of Norman Cousins and the power of therapeutic humor—using laughter and a comic perspective. And so, although I was shocked and stunned from the diagnosis, with no support system, because I had read an excerpt from Norman Cousins's book* Anatomy of an Illness *when I was in college, I ran to the video store and got every standup comedy tape they had.*

Fighting back tears and holding on to her tall stack of videotapes, Saranne went home to face her young daughter. After relieving the babysitter, she fed, bathed, and tucked Lauriel into bed as fast as she could, knowing that she would not be able to hold back her tears for very long. As soon as she closed the door to her daughter's room, Saranne went into the other room and collapsed into sobs. How would she go in for treatment? Who would help her? How would she earn a living? Who would take her daughter to school on treatment days? These questions raced through her mind in a vicious loop. Then, after a long while, she looked over at her pile of videotapes and saw Eddie Murphy staring back at her.

> *I said, "Look, it worked for Norman Cousins. Let's see if it can work for me." And so, I put in Eddie Murphy, and at first, I*

was hysterically crying. I couldn't hear the jokes, couldn't hear the punch lines, couldn't hear the laughter. But I just kept repeating, "It worked for Norman Cousins, maybe it can work for me." And eventually I started to catch the punch lines and eventually I started to laugh. And then I got hysterically laughing. And I realized that the line between comedy and trauma is so fine. So fine! Tears of sadness and tears of joy have two different compositions, but they're still tears and still cathartic.

Having this experience made Saranne realize that switching from trauma to laughter would not be as hard as she had thought—and perhaps Norman Cousins had been onto something. As she watched the videos, she noticed that an intense bout of laughter seemed to short-circuit all her trauma and fear. So, she stayed up that entire night watching every single video she had rented. By the time her daughter awoke the next morning, Saranne was clear about what she needed to do. She and her daughter purposefully had to create an environment of joy and laughter in order to balance out all the fear and side effects that were coming their way:

I said to my daughter, "We are going to make an appointment to laugh every day." And she said, "Is that like a play date?" [laughs] And I was like "Yeah!" Then I said, "And you're going to be my humor buddy. Every day we're going to make each other laugh at this appointment to laugh." And she said, "Is that like a playmate, Mommy?" And I was like "Yeah!" And then it hit me—out of the mouth of babes. I mean, what happened? How did I lose my playmates? And how did those play dates stop? From the divorce and moving, and we had a fire, and the stress of earning a living—just even raising a child—and having sick family members. All these stressors just kind of sucked the

consistent joy and fun out of my life. I mean, no wonder I had
cancer!

So, Saranne asked her daughter to help her make a list of all the things that made them laugh. Her daughter's suggestions included making funny sounds and faces, dressing up, dancing, and telling jokes. Saranne had to pause again when she heard such simple wisdom coming out of her daughter's mouth. As an adult, Saranne had lost so many of the simple pleasures in life. Now that she was facing stage 4 breast cancer, she was determined not only to get them back, but never to lose them again:

We made a commitment that every day, twice a day—once in
the morning and once in the evening—we were going to take a
minute and really have fun. And what we realized was that it
was like working out at a gym—the more we exercised laughter,
fun, joy, and playfulness, the more it permeated our days. And as
we were going through this, everybody was like "Wow! You and
your daughter are so happy! [The treatment] is killing your body,
but look at you guys! You dance through life together!" People
started asking us . . . "What is your secret? How are you doing
this?"

When Saranne had recovered from her initial surgery and was preparing to start chemotherapy for the first time, she decided she wanted to throw a Chemo Comedy Party for herself. So, she brought sparkling cider, party favors, and little hors d'oeuvres to the hospital. She wanted it to be as festive as a birthday party, a true celebration of life. At first, some people were skeptical, even offended. "What's so funny about cancer?" they asked. However, by the end of her six-hour chemotherapy treatment, nearly everyone had joined in on the fun—doctors, nurses, family members, patients, and even pharmaceutical reps. As she looked around at all the smiling faces from her chemo chair, she realized this party was just as joyful as any party she might have thrown at her home. And in that moment, she had an epiphany:

> *It was in the middle of that chemo treatment that I realized my life's mission. It came to me in a flash: we were supposed to start an organization called The ComedyCures Foundation. The phone number would be 1-888-HA-HA-HA-HA. We would bring joy, humor, a comedic perspective, and hope to the trenches of treatment, and we would help patients discover—and family members and support givers and medical caregivers—we would help them* all *realize that you can reframe this medical situation, that you can rebuild your life even though you're in the middle of this crisis. You can rebuild a life that is much more infused with good things like hope, joy, laughter, fun, and play.*

Later that evening, while resting between bouts of vomiting from the chemotherapy, Saranne wrote out the details of her vision for The ComedyCures Foundation on her bed with her head in a trash can. That piece of paper turned out to be her guiding light over the next two and a half years, allowing her to focus on something other than all the treatment she was enduring.

During her intensive Western medical treatment, which included two more surgeries, forty-four radiation treatments, and almost nonstop chemotherapy, Saranne used a variety of mental, emotional, and spiritual techniques to help get her through the ordeal. One of them was following her intuition, which told her to eliminate all sources of hatred and anger from her life and release suppressed emotions from her past. Saranne began to spend less time with people she felt were negative or, in her words, "parasitic" and more time with people who made her laugh and feel loved. Much to her surprise, this quickly led to a very noticeable change: at the end of each day she felt recharged instead of drained. This new surge of energy allowed her to rebuild her life with only positive values, such as health, fairness, and happiness.

Hearing about how much Saranne was changing her life made me remember her earlier comment of "No wonder I had cancer." Therefore, I asked Saranne if she had any thoughts as to what might cause cancer. She immediately replied:

> *I do think that there are environmental issues, of course, like decreasing sugar, eating less hormonal products, not living near a power plant, not smoking, etc. But in my case, and in other cases that I'm privy to, so much of it was about unprocessed pain, trauma, and hate. Once I started to deal with those disappointments, those fears, and to remove the toxic people out of my life, my cancer didn't really have a stranglehold on me anymore.*

After she was done cleaning up her negative relationships with other people, Saranne next turned her attention to her relationship with God. She had been spiritual before her diagnosis, but once cancer came into her life, Saranne actively started a dialogue with God:

> *I really looked at it as, I wouldn't have gotten cancer unless I was supposed to see something or help this world in a way that I would never be able to do if I wasn't put in that situation. And so, instead of ever saying "Why me?" I actually always said, "Okay, I'm listening. What am I supposed to learn here, or what*

*am I supposed to teach here? How is my cancer journey supposed
to help make the world better? What impact am I supposed to
have in that chemo chair that I would never have known about if
I hadn't gotten cancer?"*

In this way, Saranne felt empowered by her cancer diagnosis as
opposed to victimized by it. Instead of becoming angry with God,
she spent her time looking for signs and clues as to what she was
supposed to be doing differently with her life. Treating God as if
he were her chief medical adviser, Saranne simply tried to listen—
deeply listen—for divine guidance. When she listened in this way,
answers usually came to her quite clearly:

> *I realized that my cancer was a wake-up call—that my cancer,
> and the pain behind that cancer, was just part of a journey
> that had to happen. So that when I was faced with all of the
> challenges of being told, "You have cancer. You have less than
> five years to live. Your cancer is not responding [to treatment],"
> I could stand up to that diagnosis and say, "Says who?! I'm not
> going to buy it! I am not going to ingest that and play that drama
> out. I have enough strength and focus, enough discipline and
> reasons to live, that I'll figure this out with God's help. And if I
> look at this as a wake-up call to focus my vision somewhere, then
> I don't need to die. I just need to meet the call."*

Saranne's most powerful reason for living was her daughter,
Lauriel. With both her mother and grandmother now deceased,
Saranne wanted nothing more than to be able to raise her child. Because of this, Saranne was willing to try "anything and everything"
to get well, no matter how crazy it sounded, and her positive, open-
minded attitude allowed her to see every new suggestion as a reason

to feel excited and hopeful as opposed to feeling overwhelmed. So, whether a friend's brother knew a healer, someone's uncle was an acupuncturist, or a neighbor was making some kind of special herbal brew, Saranne enthusiastically tried anything that was suggested to her in the hopes of "waking up her immune system." This included changing to a macrobiotic diet, although that did not seem to curb her cancer very much, so she then tried to eat plenty of vegetables, legumes, and healthy proteins while also limiting sugar, refined grains, red meat, coffee, and alcohol. Underlying all these choices was an unwavering belief that eventually one of them would work:

> *I believe also that it was the faith that at any minute this cancer could go away. . . . Once I started to research and look for other people who have had a spontaneous remission or a miracle, I realized that this isn't so unusual. Just not so unusual! And why us? Why did we get this blessing [of Radical Remission]? What I've realized is I listened for it. I listened for this blessing. I* hear *it! I hear "Go see this doctor." I hear "Take this treatment." I hear to make sure that I'm injecting joy and total gratitude into each moment. I think it's more about listening. I think we don't listen. We're so bombarded with stimulation we don't actually take time to listen to our bodies. And I listen. I hear it.*

At this point in Saranne's cancer journey, most people would have been frustrated by the lack of progress they were experiencing. For two and a half years now she had been on a constant cycle of surgery, chemotherapy, and radiation, as well as any alternative treatment that was suggested to her, and yet her cancer continued to grow at every turn. However, thanks to her commitment to find at least some amount of joy in each day, she was able to remain positive and hopeful that things could still turn around at any moment. And then, one day, they did.

Saranne was busy preparing for a fourth, potentially life-threatening surgery during her third year of treatment when her phone starting ringing off the hook. Apparently, the Dalai Lama's doctor—a man named Yeshi Dhonden—had been featured that night on the TV show *Dateline NBC* regarding his Tibetan herbal treatment for late-stage cancer patients. Though Saranne had not seen the show, many of her friends had, and they were all calling to tell her that she simply *had* to go see him.

As you might imagine, nearly everyone who watched the show that night was trying to make an appointment to see Dr. Dhonden, so Saranne was one of thousands who were added to his waiting list. Nevertheless, with her persistent optimism guiding her, she decided to ask absolutely everyone she met if they could somehow help her see the Dalai Lama's doctor. Everywhere she went, everyone she talked to, she asked if they had any sort of connection to Dr. Dhonden. After a few months of doing this, while talking to a newly diagnosed patient about ComedyCures and its strategies for living with cancer, Saranne's positive persistence finally paid off. This person had an "in" with Dr. Dhonden's people and offered to make an appointment for Saranne. This was only a few days before her scheduled surgery:

> *I was told to bring my urine, go to New York City while fasting, and meet the Dalai Lama's doctor. He had no records; he had no reports on me. I sat with him, knee to knee. He felt my pulse. And he scrunched his face up, very confused. And then he laughed. And I laughed back. And then he scrunched up his face again, and he looked at me and, through the interpreter, said, "You are very well." I had stage 4 cancer that no one could get a handle on,*

*and he's telling me I'm very well! [laughs] And I looked him in
the eye, and I said, "I know." And he said again, "You are very,
very well!" And I said, "I know!" [laughs]*

Saranne was encouraged by this healer's declaration, because the
truth was, she did feel well. She was happier than she had ever been,
because she was making happiness and joy her number one priority
each day. After this brief interaction, Dr. Dhonden began to point
to various places on her body in complete silence. Her awe began to
build as she watched him, with incredible accuracy, point to every
place on her body where she had either had cancer in the past or
had cancer presently. "He could see what scans couldn't see," she
said and was instantly hopeful that this man could help her:

*Then he scrunched his face up again and said, "This is old." And
I said, "I know." And then he said, "Can you be patient?" And
I laughed so hard, and I said, "Dr. Dhonden"—again through
the interpreter—"If I could be patient, I probably wouldn't have
cancer right now." [laughs] Then he said, "Tibetan herbs don't
work the way Western medicine does. You have to be patient and
let the herbs collect in your system. Western medicine comes in
very quickly and destroys the cells. Eastern medicine builds in
your system and creates energy in your immune system. And then
your immune system fights your own disturbance."*

Intriguingly, Yeshi Dhonden never referred to Saranne's illness
as "cancer" but only as a "disturbance" in her body. At this point,
Saranne was eager to get started on his herbs, so she asked him
what she could expect in terms of a time line. He said that while her
symptoms of cancer should start to go away in about a month, her
scans would likely not show a reduction in cancer until about three

months. Thrilled with the possibility of her cancer actually going away, Saranne's only remaining issue was cost. Much to her happy surprise, however, while her chemo had cost about twelve hundred dollars per day, the herbs would cost only about a dollar per day:

> So, he asked me if I would take his herbs. And I said, "Sir, if you asked me to hang naked off the Statue of Liberty right now and sing 'God Bless America,' I would do it." [laughs] He laughed, and then he said, "No, I just need you to take my herbs." [laughs] So, I started to take the herbs—and within thirty-six hours my most major symptoms started to dissipate. He had said it would take about a month!

Through her experience, Saranne had developed her own comprehensive list of twenty-six subtle symptoms that arose in her body whenever her cancer was growing. Even though her Western doctors did not take her unusual list of symptoms seriously, Saranne trusted what they meant for her body. Amazingly, after only a day and a half of taking Dr. Dhonden's herbs, three of her major symptoms disappeared: extreme fatigue, a burning sensation on her lips, and an internal itching and burning sensation at the site of her cancer.

This quicker-than-expected improvement gave her the courage she needed to postpone her fourth surgery and tell her Western doctors that she only wanted to take the herbs and be monitored closely. With much resistance, they agreed to her request and scanned her three weeks later. The scan showed that the rate at which her cancer was growing had slowed; however, it was still there. Trying to focus on the fact that it was at least slowing down, Saranne asked to keep going with the herbs. Her six-week scan, much to everyone's surprise, showed that the cancer had stopped growing—it was still there, but stagnant. By now, she had developed her own theory about why the herbs were working:

What the herbs did was wake up my immune system, and then my own body fought my own cancer. . . . My Western medicine treatment [had] shocked the cancer and stunned it, but then when my body recovered from the shock and stun, the cancer just came back with a bigger vengeance. It didn't cure it. No matter what chemo I tried, I was chemo-resistant. . . . Previously, [my Western doctors had] explained to me, using their hands, that my cancer was rising and my immune system was crashing. And that was because my immune system was malfunctioning to begin with, because the cancer got momentum. And then, once [the immune system] was suppressed by all the different chemotherapies, the cancer was really having a field day, and my immune system was just getting worse. When I was introduced to the herbs, the immune system woke up. . . . Then, eventually, my immune system became supercharged. So, if you switch the hands around, my immune system was rising and my cancer was on the decline.

At the three-month mark, right on track with Dr. Dhonden's prediction, Saranne's scan showed that her tumors were starting to shrink. She was overwhelmed with joy—the moment she had always believed would happen was finally happening. Over the next fifteen months, The ComedyCures Foundation flourished while her health gradually continued to improve. Then, in 2001, eighteen months after beginning the herbs, her scans showed what she had been waiting for: no evidence of disease. With a twinge of awe still in her voice, Saranne recalls the fateful words of her oncologist that day: "Do *not* stop what you're doing."

Saranne has not stopped—in any way, shape, or form. As someone who never needed much sleep to begin with, she now uses her boundless energy to work day and night on her ever-expanding foundation. Among other things, the foundation brings top-notch comedians in to entertain hospital patients at numerous free Laughing Luncheons. Saranne also advises cancer patients on how to redesign their lives from a joyous, laughter-filled perspective, just as she did when she was sick. Even if their bodies do not experience the kind of Radical Remission hers did, she still feels good knowing that she helped to improve their emotional and spiritual quality of life. Finally, she continues to take her daily dose of both laughter and herbs:

> *If I sense any of my cancer symptoms are recurring, I just meet*
> *with or write Yeshi Dhonden's team and they change the herbs,*
> *and we watch to see if my body responds, and traditionally it*
> *does. The one or two times over the years where I didn't feel the*
> *decrease of symptoms over time, he changed the herbs again.*
> *And so we just stay ahead of [the cancer] by keeping my immune*
> *system really functioning at a very high level.*

While some people will look at Saranne's story and think that the Tibetan herbs alone caused her remission, she disagrees. In her opinion, it was the multifaceted healing approach she took *before* meeting Dr. Dhonden that led him to say to her "You are *very* well":

> *I often get asked, "Do you* really *think comedy cures?" And*
> *what I always say is that comedy cured my spirit and gave me*
> *the strength to fight the physical battle. I had the knowledge of*
> *the life and teachings and research of Norman Cousins. I had*
> *something to latch on to that first weekend that was positive, and*

I researched more and more about the power of the mind over the body, and especially the power of joy and hope over the body. So, I don't believe that it was just one element that helped me to have a Radical Remission and heal. I believe that, because my mind and my spirit were so strong, and [because] I created an environment—emotionally, spiritually, medically, societally— that was so full, so abundant, so healthy, so joyful . . . when my immune system did wake up [due to the herbs], the rest of my body was ready to follow.

Today, more than thirteen years after being diagnosed with stage 4 breast cancer, Saranne is still cancer-free, now happily remarried with three kids, and thrilled to be alive to witness her singer/song-writer daughter, Lauriel, get ready to release her first album.

———————

SARANNE IS A wonderful example of someone who used conventional medicine at the same time as complementary techniques in order to strengthen her body, mind, and spirit. This multi-faceted healing approach not only helped her endure the many years of arduous medical treatment, but it also gave Saranne other options—such as daily laughter therapy and Tibetan herbs—when her chemo, surgery, and radiation stopped working. No matter how sick or afraid she may have felt on any given day, she did not allow herself to go to sleep without at least five minutes of laughter or happiness. In her opinion, it was this daily habit that allowed her body, mind, and spirit to stay alive during her years of intense medical treatment.

Action Steps

Many cancer patients—as well as many people who simply hope to prevent cancer—will read a story like Saranne's and doubt that they could create happiness in their lives every day, much less while in the midst of a life-threatening illness. The ugly truth is that many of us are *not* happy—twenty million Americans suffer from some form of depression each year.[9] What's worse is that millions more are not clinically depressed, yet are deeply bored and unsatisfied with their lives. These emotional states also do nothing to help our immune systems fight off illnesses.

The good news is that, as Saranne discovered, it does not take much effort to bring a bit of happiness into your life, even when you're in the middle of a traumatic cancer journey. It does, however, require consistency, such as Saranne's daily appointment to laugh with her daughter. Just as you won't get physically fit sitting on your couch, you won't increase your happiness by doing nothing. Instead, you have to purposefully try to do things each day that might bring you some amount of happiness or joy. It may feel forced at first, but if you continue with your daily commitment to happiness, the serotonin will soon start flowing more quickly and easily.

Here are some simple suggestions that many Radical Remission survivors have tried in order to increase their positive emotions:

A Prescription for Fun

- *Start every day with a smile or a feeling of gratitude.* To smile, start your day by watching your favorite YouTube video, subscribing to a Joke of the Day e-mail service, or flipping through a photo album (actual or electronic) that makes you smile. Or, to feel gratitude, keep a gratitude journal by your bed and write down five things that you're grateful for before getting up each morning.

- *Monitor your media.* These days, we are bombarded with a constant stream of information, most of it negative and fear inducing. Make sure that you either smile or feel gratitude *before* reading or watching the news each day, and experiment with reducing the amount of news you take in. By doing so, you may notice a shift in your emotions for the better, while still being able to stay up on current events.

- *Examine your entertainment.* In addition to the news, take a look at the TV shows and movies you watch. Detective dramas and murder mysteries can be thrilling, but they won't boost your body's immune system the way a comedy does; instead, they often activate a stress response in the body. Therefore, try to add at least one more comedic show to your entertainment roster each week.

- *Find fun friends.* Just as alarming news and dramatic entertainment can turn on your body's stress response instead of your healing response, so can family and friends. So, just as Saranne did, take a hard look at your relationships and ask yourself, "Do I feel energized or drained by this person?" Start to limit the amount of time you spend with people who drain you, and increase the amount of time you spend with those who energize you.

- *Get active.* Find activities that bring you joy and that you can do in your daily life right now. Some examples may include exercising, walking outside in nature, gardening, singing, dancing, meditating, taking photographs, cooking, calling an old friend, giving someone a present, joining a local chorus, taking music lessons, or volunteering. Make a commitment to do an actual activity (watching TV doesn't count) that brings you joy at least three times per week.

If you are one of the many people who have lost touch with what brings you joy, take out a piece of paper and write down all the times you remember feeling happy, even if they were a very long time ago. Then examine the list and ask yourself, "Which of these things do I want to start doing again?" If you can't do them for some reason (e.g., you are too sick to travel), try to think of another activity that will give you a similar feeling of happiness. For example, instead of traveling, you could make a commitment to try out a new restaurant or local event each week.

- *Do a nightly check-in.* Before going to sleep each night, ask yourself, "Did I have at least one moment of happiness today?" If so, make a mental note of that moment and be grateful for it. If not, reread the first suggestion and try to either smile or feel grateful before going to bed.

The life-affirming message from this chapter is actually very simple: if you are under chronic stress, your body cannot heal itself; if you instead commit to at least five minutes of happiness per day, you will provide rocket fuel to your immune system. I personally try to find moments of love, joy, and happiness daily, and I strongly urge you to do the same, because feeling happy each day—even if just for five minutes—is just as important for your health as any medicine you could ever take.

CHAPTER 7

EMBRACING SOCIAL SUPPORT

In poverty and other misfortunes of life, true friends are a sure refuge.
—ARISTOTLE

Humans are social creatures by nature, and I do not just mean that we like to get together and chat in order to blow off some steam. At a fundamental level, humans need each other to survive. This begins when we are babies. A human baby is one of the most helpless mammals on the planet, depending entirely on its mother for survival for not just months but years; in contrast, a baby horse learns how to walk in the first five minutes of life. Humans continue to depend on one another throughout their entire lives, because banding together has historically improved both our personal safety and food production.

However, the support of others is perhaps never more vital than when we are sick. Ideally, when we are ill, loved ones will be there to care for us—to make us hot soup, cover us with a blanket, and call our bosses to let them know we can't come in to work. These are the practical ways in which friends and family support us when we are not feeling well. However, researchers have recently discovered that loved ones also help our bodies in a more sophisticated way. When we are surrounded by loved ones or even our pets, the feeling of being loved releases a flood of potent hormones into our bloodstreams,[1] which not only makes us feel better emotionally but also strengthens our immune systems significantly.[2] Receiving love from others when we are sick actually helps the body heal itself.

This is why it is no surprise that receiving love from others—"social support"—turns out to be one of the nine key factors of my Radical Remission research. This chapter will explore the importance of social support in depth, focusing on its three main aspects. While we all instinctively understand the importance of support, we'll also look at the research that backs this up. We will then discover the healing story of Kathryn, a woman who never could have overcome her advanced liver cancer without the love and support she received from others. The chapter concludes with some simple steps you can take to bring more love and support into your life.

RECEIVING LOVE HELPS THE BODY HEAL

Virtually all the Radical Remission survivors I study believe that the love they received from others when they were sick actually helped their physical bodies heal. For some people, this was a surprise; they were not expecting love to have a tangible effect on their bodies. For others, the surprise was the *amount* of love unexpectedly showered upon them, not only by close friends and family but also by long-lost friends or sometimes even people they barely knew.

One such survivor is Nancy McKay, a devoted wife, mother, and minister. Nancy was fifty-four when metastatic melanoma was discovered in her lymph nodes, and her doctors told her she had only one to two years to live. Refusing to accept that prognosis, she instead put together an integrative plan that combined surgery and experimental cancer vaccines with prayer and Chinese herbs. What she was not expecting, though, was the outpouring of love she received:

An old friend recently asked me, "To what do you attribute your healing?" I saw myself reflected in his eyes and replied, "Love, prayer, and good experimental medicine." He smiled as his mind turned over what I said. Then he followed up with, "In that order?" Now I took a minute. Then I nodded, "Yes, in that order." The love came from many directions—my husband held me, my daughter offered to become pregnant right away so I might see a grandchild before I died, every person in the church where I was pastor for ten years wrote or called, a soft scarf arrived from across the country with a note that said, "Let this be the loving touch across the miles," and of course, our two cats took turns snuggling with me on the couch, never leaving me alone. At my lowest moments, a sense of warmth and caring flowed around me. I learned that I could never again say I wasn't loved. I got it. I am loved—even by me.

It has now been more than twenty years since Nancy's doctors told her she had only a year or two left to live, and she is currently enjoying a love-filled, cancer-free life. In a similar vein, many of the alternative healers I interview also believe that sending love to someone who is sick can significantly improve that person's physical state. One of those healers is Dane Silva, a kahuna healer from Hawaii who provided this vignette about sending love to patients:

I walked in just in time to hear the doctor tell my patient, "You're going to die tonight unless you give me permission to hook you up to these machines." It was to keep her heart beating and her lungs moving. And she would not give him permission. So, on his way out I stopped him and I said, "Are there any other options or alternatives?" He said, "Oh, no. If she doesn't give me permission to hook her up to these machines, she will die tonight." I said, "Well, you know, I called a whole bunch of friends to come over tonight and we believe there's another option." Two hours later, I left; I went home. All the friends were there, singing, telling jokes, playing music, having a lot of fun. The next morning, she left. *She went to rehab and returned home. There was another alternative. She did not go on the machines. When I left, there she was, breathing normally and her heart rate was good and her oxygen saturation levels were almost perfect. . . . The family members, the loved ones, provided that energy for that psychosocial healing.*

From Dane's point of view as a kahuna healer, love is a high-frequency, health-inducing form of energy. Therefore, giving love—or high-frequency energy—to a sick person is believed to help that person clear out any energetic blockages and help restore balance to his or her bodily systems.

Scientifically, there is a large body of evidence to support the idea that receiving emotional love from others is beneficial to the physical body. First, from a more general standpoint, studies have repeatedly shown that people with more social connections live significantly longer than people with fewer social connections,[3] and they also have lower cancer rates.[4] What's so amazing about this health-giving force of social connection is that it has been shown to be more beneficial than exercise, diet, or even drinking and smoking.[5] In other words, close-knit communities that regularly eat and relax together live longer than average, even if they eat fatty foods, drink alcohol, smoke, or don't exercise much. (Obviously, if you are trying to be the healthiest you can be, you will work on increasing your social support network while also eating healthfully, reducing alcohol and tobacco consumption, and exercising.)

If you are dealing with a cancer diagnosis, the good news is that strong social connections have been shown to significantly lengthen your survival time as well—by an average of 25 percent.[6] In one recent study, breast cancer patients who were able to increase their social support during their cancer journeys reduced their risk of dying by an incredible 70 percent.[7] If you are single with cancer, don't worry. You do not need to be married or have kids in order to benefit from the healing effect of social support. Rather, studies have shown that having strong social support is what matters most, and it doesn't matter whether that strong support is obtained from two close friends, thirty acquaintances, or one spouse.[8]

In addition to these broader studies, which observe the survival rates of large groups of people, researchers have looked into what happens inside an individual's body when he or she receives love and support from friends and family. What they have found—through brain MRIs, blood tests, and saliva analysis—is that receiving love and social support leads to significant increases in powerful healing hormones, such as dopamine, oxytocin, serotonin, and endorphins.[9] These hormones in turn boost the immune system by sending signals to decrease inflammation, increase blood and oxygen circulation, and increase the number of white blood cells, red blood cells, helper T cells, and natural killer cells.[10] All these changes help your body find and remove cancer cells. What these studies show us is what Radical Remission survivors and alternative healers already believe is true: receiving love from others helps your body heal.

THE GOAL IS NOT TO FEEL ALONE

The second aspect of receiving love and support is the idea that the overall goal is not to feel alone, although the methods for achieving this will vary from person to person. For example, some cancer patients need only to be surrounded by their close family and friends in order not to feel alone. For other patients, friends and family may provide some comfort, but they may still feel alone on their cancer journeys. These people will typically benefit from joining cancer support groups or group exercise classes for cancer patients, in order to connect with others going through a similar experience.

Many of the Radical Remission survivors I talk to tend to want to be around cancer patients making choices similar to theirs. They work on not feeling alone by reading as many Radical Remission cases as they can find or trying to meet Radical Remission survivors in person whenever possible. Then again, some people I counsel are best able not to feel alone when they *are* alone, such as when they are in deep prayer or meditation. Regardless of the variety of ways in which to accomplish it, the common goal is simply not to feel alone.

"Rita," a librarian who was diagnosed with stage 4 non-Hodgkin's MALT (mucosa-associated lymphoid tissue) lymphoma, found multiple ways of not feeling alone. Among other things, she immediately sought out a support group:

> *I joined support groups because I've read that going to a support group increases your longevity—and just as a way to let out a lot of things that you wouldn't really be able to talk about to other people without them thinking of you as a cancer subject. . . . That's also why I wanted to continue to be a health librarian, because I felt that, from people I've met who have their own [healing] stories, I've been able to benefit from understanding what happens when you have cancer and what happens when you're in a situation where things are relatively unknown—how people cope and things like that.*

During the three months it took Rita to get a second and third opinion from other doctors, and while she was working diligently to increase her social support and reduce her stress, her lymphoma went away almost entirely. Both Rita and her doctor were shocked by this sudden turn of events. Since then, she continues to maintain a good level of social support—and her cancer has continued to remain in remission for more than eight years.

Many of the healers I study similarly emphasize the danger of loneliness to a person's health. For example, Atarangi Muru, a traditional Maori healer from New Zealand, considers loving support from one's community to be part of the basic definition of health:

Health for most Maori can be [defined as] how their whānau [families] are thriving, the balance one has in life, what they do for their local community, the influence of our elders in our lives, and how happy and balanced our children are. . . . Modern [Maori health] maintenance is done mostly through tribal gatherings, like our kapa haka *[dramatic performances],* waka ama *[outrigger canoe races], and local sports. Very few Maori go for individual sports; they tend to choose more group settings.*

The Maori believe that being part of a strongly bonded community is healing for the body. When I was conducting research in New Zealand, I was struck by how closely bonded the Maori were and how they all lived near one another in tight-knit communities. This is quite different from typical American culture, where we tend to live in fenced-off houses and often do not know our neighbors. The Maori healers I met view this kind of behavior as strange, lonely, and ultimately unhealthy, because it means you receive very little healing energy from other people.

The Maori may be right to think of us as strange, since studies have repeatedly shown that loneliness or a lack of social connection does, in fact, lead to an earlier death;[11] in some cases, loneliness has been shown to increase your chances of dying by as much as 50 percent.[12] In one very large study on breast cancer patients, women who had the fewest social connections before their breast cancer diagnoses were *twice* as likely to die of breast cancer than women who started off with strong social connections. What's even scarier is that the women in this study who continued to go through their cancer journeys alone ended up being four times as likely to die of breast cancer compared to women who gained the support of ten or more friends.[13] And when researchers tested the blood and saliva of lonely people, they found that loneliness is associated with increased cortisol levels (the stress hormone)[14] and a depressed immune profile,[15] which means a decreased ability to remove cancer cells from the body. Taken altogether, these loneliness studies show us that just as social connection can be a powerful immune booster, loneliness can be a silent killer. Therefore, if you are feeling lonely in your life, it is just as vital to your health that you take steps to reduce your loneliness as it is to do things like eat your vegetables and exercise regularly.

THE IMPORTANCE OF PHYSICAL TOUCH

The third aspect of receiving love and support is the importance of physical touch when it comes to healing. I am not talking about sexual intimacy but rather things like hugging, putting an arm around someone's shoulder, cuddling, or giving someone a pain-relieving massage. For many of the survivors I work with, receiving regular human touch is an essential part of their healing process, especially if they are in pain or bedridden.

One such person who benefited immensely from physical touch was a woman named "Diana," who was sixty-one when she was diagnosed with stage 4 cervical cancer. She first tried conventional medicine to its fullest, going through eight rounds of various types of chemotherapy, although none of them helped. Thankfully, the emotional support and physical touch she received from her husband helped her get through this difficult journey:

> *I was in the hospital 115 days before they sent me home to die, and my husband never left my side. He slept in the room every night with me; he was there all day, every day. When I was the sickest, he crawled into bed with me to hold me. I never saw or heard of another [person] getting the support he gave me. It was so calming to me to know that he was there. It still brings tears of gratitude to my eyes when I think of how he was with me.*

Diana was eventually sent home on hospice care, at which time she asked all her friends and family to pray for her while she surrendered fully to God's will. Amazingly, her health slowly turned around, and now, more than five years later, she has no evidence of disease. She is especially grateful for all the physical comfort, emotional support, and prayers she received from her family and friends.

One of the healers I met who uses gentle, physical touch in her work is Pamela Miles, a Reiki master practicing since 1986. Reiki is a spiritual healing practice originating in Japan that involves offering gentle, healing touch to a person who is fully clothed. The hand placements are noninvasive on the head, front and back of the torso, and anywhere the client has a complaint. This gentle laying on of hands elicits a natural healing response in the patient's body. Pamela describes the power of Reiki touch this way:

> *Although we don't yet know why or how this happens, Reiki touch somehow enhances the patient's sense of spiritual connectedness, bringing an awareness that while we live as individuals, we are also each part of something larger than our separate beings. Feel-*

ing a spiritual connection allows your system to let go of its habit-ual holding patterns and drop into deep relaxation. In this state, your system's self-healing mechanisms recalibrate themselves, so that the body can more effectively address areas that have become unbalanced through stress.

In terms of the studies conducted on human touch, research has shown that human-to-human contact releases many of the same healing hormones that are released when we receive love and sup-port (e.g., serotonin, dopamine, endorphins), although oxytocin—known colloquially as the "cuddle" hormone—is secreted in particularly large amounts as a result of physical touch.[16] Oxytocin is a powerful hormone that helps the body in numerous ways: it re-duces inflammation and pain, decreases blood pressure and cortisol levels, improves digestion (and therefore the absorption of nutri-ents), and—perhaps most relevant for cancer patients—improves immune function.[17] This amazing list of oxytocin's health benefits explains why so many of the people I research emphasize the impor-tance of physical touch when it comes to healing.

If you aren't in a cuddling relationship at the moment, not to worry—a pet will do just as well. Studies have shown that we re-ceive the same, wonderful release of healing hormones from being around pets as we do from being around our friends and family, and pet owners have been shown to live significantly longer than non-pet owners.[18] One of my favorite pet studies involved two groups of rabbits that were both fed high-cholesterol diets, but only one group received a daily petting session from humans. At the end of the study, the rabbits who had received daily petting had 60 per-cent less blockage in their arteries than the rabbits who were left in isolation[19]—in other words, physical touch allowed these animals to better eliminate all that excess cholesterol they were being forced to eat. In human studies, researchers have found that hugging for only ten seconds a day can lower your blood pressure, reduce cortisol, and increase oxytocin[20]—so, in addition to your apple a day, you may want to consider a hug or two a day.

———

NOW THAT WE have explored the main aspects of social support, I'd like to share with you Kathryn's story. Despite the wide variety of things Kathryn Alexander did to help heal her cancer, she feels with absolute certainty that her recovery never would have happened without the tremendous love and support she received from her friends and church community. Her story is a beautiful example of the healing power not only of giving but also—and perhaps more important—of receiving.

—❧ **Kathryn's Story** ❧—

Kathryn Alexander was sixty-three when she fainted on her way to the bathroom one morning. As a single (divorced), self-employed woman living on her own, no one was there to help. Luckily, she awoke only a few minutes later, feeling very disoriented and with a throbbing bump on her head. Because she had never fainted before, she immediately called the triage nurse at the local hospital, and the nurse advised her to find someone to drive her to the emergency room, just to be sure that it was nothing more serious than dehydration.

Kathryn was a bit reluctant to go, because she could not afford individual health insurance at the time and was therefore waiting for Medicare to start at age sixty-five. However, she decided that fainting was not something to take lightly, so she called a friend who willingly offered to drive her to the nearby emergency room.

A close-knit group of friends and her strong church community were her primary sources of support at this time, because she was no longer in contact with her ex-husband, and her only daughter lived over a thousand miles away.

Unfortunately, what started off as a minor fainting spell turned into the biggest health challenge of Kathryn's life when a precautionary CT scan revealed a large tumor on her liver. She spent a week in the hospital, with the bills mounting every day, as the doctors tried to figure out exactly what was wrong with her. The indicators for liver cancer were slightly elevated in her blood, which, combined with the large tumor on her CT scan, led her doctors to recommend immediate surgery in order to remove the possibly cancerous tumor. The surgery would require them to remove one-half to two-thirds of her liver; however, this is not quite as dangerous as it sounds, because the liver is the only organ in the human body that has the ability to regenerate.

Kathryn, however, felt intuitively that the surgery was too rash of a decision; she wanted to be sure it was cancer before removing possibly two-thirds of her liver. So, she insisted first on a biopsy, which would involve only a minor surgical procedure. She asked for recommendations for a surgeon who could perform this biopsy, and one doctor's name kept coming up over and over again. He was currently out of town, though, so Kathryn was released from the hospital with an appointment to see him a week later. When she met him, she told him about her wish for a biopsy before having such major surgery:

I said [to the surgeon] that I wanted a biopsy, and he said, "Fine," and so we scheduled the biopsy, which was supposed to be an outpatient procedure. I called the hospital a day before the biopsy was scheduled to ask how long I would be in there, so that I could tell somebody what time to pick me up. And she said,

*"Two weeks." And I said, "For a biopsy?!" She went to check,
and he had scheduled the surgery without telling me—because in
a surgeon's mind, a biopsy is just a preliminary to surgery. They
just do it to figure out what to do. So, I canceled that! And I did
finally get a biopsy [from a different doctor].*

When Kathryn received her biopsy results, the news was not
good: she had stage 3B hepatocellular (liver) cancer, and her tumor
was the size of a grapefruit. A cloud of heaviness immediately settled
around her. Her worst-case scenario had arrived, and the possibility
of an earlier-than-expected death was now staring her in the face:

*I remember standing by the window [of the hospital room] and
being asked whether I wanted to live or not. And I said, "Yes.
I want to live." . . . I was really clear that I didn't feel complete
[in life], and so I had no intentions of wanting to leave [this life]
incompletely. I'm not afraid of death . . . but I just didn't feel
it was the time. . . . So, I knew then and there I would not die.
And there is a place that you come from when you make that
choice. It's not about words. It's not about thoughts. It's truly
from your core being. You're clear that that's exactly what's going
to happen.*

Once Kathryn had decided to live, however, she next had to deal
with one of life's most pressing issues: money. As an adjunct college professor with no benefits, she was continually living month
to month off her small teaching income. She was only two years
away from receiving health insurance through Medicare, but in the
meantime, it had simply been too expensive for her to purchase individual health insurance. So, while her soul had chosen to live, her
mind was worried about how to pay for it:

One of the things that I said when I had that conversation in the hospital room was—because I had no insurance, and I had no idea what to do—so, I said, "If I'm going to survive this, it's because other people care." And people showed up! I mean I couldn't work. I had no savings. I had no insurance. But somehow it all worked. And it worked because I was able to share the reality of my experience, and people resonated with that, and they just stepped in to do whatever was needed.

As soon as word got around to Kathryn's friends and church community that she had stage 3 liver cancer, she was flooded by an instant tidal wave of support, both financial and emotional. One person, who was really only an acquaintance at the time, told Kathryn that she would give Kathryn her monthly rent money for as long as she needed. With tears in her eyes, Kathryn gratefully accepted, because she knew that she would have to stop teaching for a while in order to focus fully on her health. She had also done a lot of fund-raising for her church in the past, so her church community returned the favor by organizing a fund-raiser in her honor, the funds from which helped pay her exorbitant hospital bills. The financial support that came in continued to humble and amaze her:

I had a friend who was talking about me to people he knew, and somebody that he knew sent me a thousand dollars. And I have never met the man! I didn't know him, didn't know of him, never met him. . . . The lesson here is that we are loved not for who we are, but because we are. He didn't know me. He wasn't giving to me personally, because he didn't know me personally. He was giving because he cared for another human being.

This kind of anonymous generosity filled Kathryn with immense gratitude and humility—and a growing sense that she was loved. At the request of her friends, she also started sending out e-mail updates about what was going on with her. The point of these e-mails was to keep her friends and church community up to date on her status. However, she was always amazed by the unexpected responses of love and support she received after sending out an e-mail. The replies of emotional encouragement were especially poignant, and she kept all the responses in a folder on her computer so she could go back and reread them whenever she needed an emotional lift.

In addition to making her feel loved and taken care of, the emotional and financial support she received allowed her to follow the path of healing that intuitively felt right to her. Even though she now officially had cancer, her long background in complementary medicine told her that surgically removing the tumor and receiving chemotherapy and radiation would not permanently solve the problem. The very idea of poisoning the organ responsible for detoxifying the body as a healing strategy dumbfounded her. Therefore, Kathryn told her doctors that she was going to try other approaches.

Even in the arena of alternative medicine, social support continued to play a key role for Kathryn. Every friend she talked to had a suggestion for a particular vitamin or herbal supplement she should try, or a particular treatment she should look into. Based on these recommendations, as well as her own research into the things they were suggesting, she tried a variety of supplements and then kept taking only the ones that made a noticeable difference in her body. One of these was an aloe supplement called Ambrotose, and another was a rice-bran supplement called Vital PSP. Meanwhile, her diet was already very healthy, so she decided not to drive herself crazy with any overly strict dietary changes:

The thought of changing my diet was more than I could deal with. I've not felt that I've eaten badly, anyway. I don't eat white flour. I don't eat white sugar. I'm mostly vegetarian—I only eat chicken. I use mostly organics and all of that, so I just didn't want to go there. I could have gone macrobiotic. I have a friend who cured herself of breast cancer with macrobiotics. In fact, I've known several people who've done that. I just couldn't do the macrobiotic diet. It's much too severe—takes more discipline than I have.

While Kathryn's intuition was not pushing her to make big dietary changes, it was telling her to try energetic healing modalities such as BodyTalk, which she tried and found incredibly helpful. One of her friends suggested that she take advantage of the free acupuncture offered by student interns at a local acupuncture college, so she also started getting acupuncture weekly. She serendipitously heard about her most important energetic treatment from a business group to which she belonged: it was a frequency healing treatment offered in Arizona called the Life Vessel:

The approach of [the Life Vessel] is a frequency approach. [The inventor] created a box that you lie in, and then you hear music and the box vibrates to the music. So, you're in a very complete space. Your entire body is vibrating at the same level of frequencies of music, and the theory, of course, is that healthy cells vibrate at a certain level, and unhealthy cells vibrate at a different level. So, if you change the vibration to health, then that which is not healthy sort of, well, disappears.

The Life Vessel treatments go along with what we have heard in some of the previous chapters about how all things in life vibrate at the atomic level. Many alternative healers use this fact as the basis for their cancer treatments, using hands-on energy healing, music therapy, or electronic machines to try to shift their patients' cells toward a healthier vibration. Such frequency treatments are currently difficult to study using today's scientific, diagnostic tools; in other words, we do not currently have the right "microscope" to see what is actually happening during these treatments. However, I hope within a few decades we will have developed the technology to evaluate this intriguing new method of treatment.

Although it was expensive, Kathryn determined that the Life Vessel was her best choice, and she was amazed by how good she felt after only one treatment. Her friends also noticed an improvement. However, the treatments were not only expensive but also required her to travel to Arizona one week a month, while being very restful the other three weeks of the month. Kathryn figured this would be impossible, but once her friends found out that she wanted to continue with the treatments, they miraculously made it happen with impromptu fund-raisers and generous financial support. Kathryn was overwhelmed with gratitude that she was being given the gift of being able to focus all her time and energy on her healing, a gift she sincerely wishes all cancer patients could receive.

Speaking of receiving, Kathryn freely admits that she was not very good at accepting help before her cancer diagnosis. She had always been the kind of person who tried to do everything herself. However, once she was diagnosed with cancer, she quickly realized that she would never be able to survive the journey if she tried to do it alone—neither financially nor emotionally. While it was difficult at first to accept so much help and support, she eventually came to view the process in a new light:

One of the biggest lessons I learned from being sick is the power of reciprocity. Reciprocity is allowing for the flow of giving and

receiving. It's giving, not manipulating or bribing or coercing.
And it's receiving, not taking or tricking. . . . And we're so used to
giving because that's a power play—it makes you feel good, like
you're "one up" and all that. But, you can't give if someone won't
receive. That was my big lesson: I had to allow for that flow. I
learned that it was a privilege for people to give, and it was also a
privilege for me to receive.

Therefore, Kathryn gratefully received the gift of the Life Vessel treatments that was given to her by her friends and church community, and she started flying down to Arizona once a month for the frequency treatment. During this time, she also saw her oncologist regularly in order to monitor her blood. Even though her visual appearance and blood work were consistently improving, her oncologist took little interest in her healing techniques:

Everybody who watched me could tell how much better I looked
when I came back [from the Life Vessel treatments]. So, I was
constantly getting feedback. And the oncologist would even say,
"You look too good to be sick." At the same time, he was trying
to get me to do chemoembolization, which I didn't do. And he
was kind of irritated that I basically wasn't taking any of his
advice. . . . He never asked me what I was doing, and when I
told him I was doing lots of stuff, he would say, "Oh, you're not
doing anything."

Even though her oncologist did not believe that what Kathryn was doing could have any real effect on her liver cancer, Kathryn knew without a doubt she was feeling healthier as a result of all the changes she was making. As a longtime believer in the mind–body connection, she also used the time she spent in the Life Vessel to meditate deeply about her life, to reflect on her past choices and emotional habits, and to ask herself why she got cancer:

I am very clear that there's a mind–body connection. . . . There was a certain situation that I was in for the fifteen years of my married life that made me very angry, but I did not truly understand it, and I didn't really know how to express the anger. . . . The anger was because I didn't feel valued. . . . And that anger lodged in my liver. I was able to see the pattern in the Life Vessel, of how I understood my experience and translated it in that way. So, I can now see how my thoughts and my feelings contributed to the sickness. And understanding that pattern doesn't mean it goes away, but it does mean that I can know it when it happens, and I can manage it now, which I couldn't before.

In Traditional Chinese Medicine theory, the liver is the organ that processes the emotion of anger. Once these mind–body insights started coming up, Kathryn decided to try to release her suppressed anger in the weeks between Life Vessel treatments. One of the many ways in which she did this was by signing up for an emotional expression class that culminated in a creative performance piece. Throughout all of this, her friends were constantly helping out or simply dropping by for a visit. Their support was a constant reminder to her that she was not alone and that other people (besides herself) wanted her to keep living. To Kathryn, this was one of the most profound aspects of her healing journey:

One of the things I truly learned [from going through cancer] is that I am valued. . . . It was a huge validation of the universe and that all life is valued. I wasn't valued because I'm me—my person, necessarily—but because my life has value. All *life has value, and that includes mine. I could no longer say, "People don't care about me."*

Feeling this outpouring of love and support from friends as well as strangers encouraged Kathryn to find that love inside herself at a more spiritual level. When I asked Kathryn if her spirituality changed in any way during her healing journey, she replied:

My philosophy about this whole process, actually, is that the whole purpose of cancer is to get people in touch with who they really are. The people that I know who have gone through [cancer] and done well have taken control and decided to be really authentic and real with themselves. They haven't said, "Oh, the doctor will cure me." Those people have not lived. So, I don't think it's so much about the method you use as it is the fact that you're in touch with who you are, which is a very spiritual place.

After eighteen months of trying this multifaceted healing approach, which involved physical, emotional, energetic, and spiritual work, the Life Vessel indicated that Kathryn's immune system was finally back to normal. It was at this point that she decided she was ready to have another CT scan. Much to her dismay, however, the scan showed that her grapefruit-size tumor had shrunk by only a tiny bit. Feeling disappointed that it was not completely gone, yet trying to trust that she had still done the right thing, Kathryn reluctantly agreed to have surgery to remove the tumor. However, what they found was not quite what anyone expected:

When my doctor opened me up, there was no more cancer in my liver—the tumor was hanging off the side of [my liver]! So, he just snipped the tumor. It ended up being minor surgery. I went home in three days! And [the surgeon] was the only doctor who ever said, "I have no idea what you are doing, but you should continue it." Again, though, he didn't ask me what I was doing.

Kathryn awoke from that minor surgery to find a room full of baffled doctors standing around her. They apparently had never seen anything like this. Kathryn, however, felt with certainty that it was the combination of love and support, Life Vessel treatments, emotional release work, and vitamin supplements that had allowed her immune system to kick into high gear and manage her cancer. It has now been more than seven years since her diagnosis of stage 3B liver cancer, and Kathryn remains healthy, happy, and above all, grateful for the love and support she received from her friends and family during those eighteen months. While the Life Vessel treatments have long since ended, her newfound ability to receive love from others is something she will keep with her always. As she puts it:

Cancer was one of the best experiences of my life. I learned so much, including one of the major ways I said no to life. I learned that people love. People love to love. It's inherent in our DNA. They look for opportunities to give, but reciprocity requires that there is a receiver for that love to flow. So, I learned how to receive love.

———————

WITHOUT ANY FAMILY nearby to help her, and because she was self-employed, Kathryn was perhaps more alone than most people are when they are diagnosed with cancer. This made it all the more important that she had a strong friend network and community to help her in her time of need. It was this support—emotional, practical, and financial—that created the foundation she needed in order to explore other complementary healing methods. None of the treatments would have been possible without the support of her friends and church community.

Action Steps

When I am counseling cancer patients, I always check in about their support network and try to brainstorm ways they can strengthen it. Many of us feel funny asking others for help because we do not want to be a burden, but as Kathryn learned so well, other people *want* to feel helpful; it is part of what makes us human. People especially want to feel helpful when someone they know or love is sick. I cannot tell you the number of friends and family members who pull me aside and tell me they want to help so badly but they just don't know how. So, here are some ideas to get you started.

If You Are a Cancer Patient

- Reach out to someone you love by picking up the phone today and just calling him or her. Simply tell that person you were thinking about him or her and wanted to know how he or she is doing. If this person doesn't know you have cancer, you do not have to tell him or her, or if this person already knows, you always have the option of telling the person that you only want to hear about how he or she is doing. People will understand that you do not want to talk about your health challenge and instead want to be distracted by non-cancer talk. Call someone else tomorrow, and repeat the process daily.

- Sign up for a gentle group exercise class in your area, or if there are exercise classes designed specifically for cancer patients, consider attending one of those.

- Join a support group of other cancer patients if that is something that appeals to you. You can try to find one through your cancer hospital, your local American Cancer Society chapter, or at the very least in an online support group. If talking with other cancer patients sounds too depressing for you, sign up for a different group activity that gets you out of the house and meeting new people, such as a photography class, a hiking club, or a bridge-playing group.

- Don't be afraid to ask for help when you need it. Your friends, family, and even acquaintances truly want to help you in any way they can, but they won't know you need help unless you ask for it. If you don't feel comfortable asking for help directly, tell a close friend what you would ideally like help with (cooking meals, running errands, social visits, etc.), and then ask him or her to e-mail your larger group of family and friends about what you need.

If You Are the Loved One of a Cancer Patient

- Call your loved one who has cancer and simply tell that person you were thinking about him or her. That is all you need to do. This person may not answer because he or she is not feeling well; in that case, leave a message that you were thinking of that person and you just wanted him or her to know. End your message by explaining that this person does not need to feel obligated to call you back. Just this one, simple action will cause a surge of healing hormones to be released throughout your sick friend's body. Try to do this at least once a week.

- Drop off healthy meals. Check in with your loved one about what he or she is eating these days (since that person may be on a restricted diet, e.g., vegan). When you can, cook a meal that goes along with this person's diet restrictions and drop it off in a freezable container.

- Offer to run errands or help with household chores. Finding the time and energy to keep up with things like grocery shopping, cleaning, and laundry can be very difficult for people as they go through their cancer journey.

- Plan a day of pampering or distraction. An afternoon at a spa or attending a leisurely sporting event are two suggestions that many cancer patients have enjoyed.

- Don't get overwhelmed thinking that you always have to do something in order to be supportive. The goal is to show your love, and a simple phone call or e-mail every couple of days telling that person you are thinking about him or her goes a very long way in boosting someone's spirits—and immune system.

———

I HOPE THIS chapter has convinced you that receiving love and support from others is as essential for your health as eating a vegetable-rich diet or taking antioxidant supplements. That's because what we feel emotionally is instantly translated into chemicals and hormones that either strengthen or weaken our immune systems. And when we feel loved and cared for by others, the rush of healing hormones released by the master glands in our brains affects our bodies in such a way that our immune systems suddenly have renewed energy to repair cells, clear out toxins, and most important, remove cancer cells. So, in addition to remembering to take your vitamins each day, don't forget to ask yourself these two questions: To whom have I given love today? And, from whom did I *receive* love?

CHAPTER 8

DEEPENING YOUR SPIRITUAL CONNECTION

The greatest mistake in the treatment of diseases is that there are physicians for the body and physicians for the soul, although the two cannot be separated.

—PLATO

Spirituality is a delicate subject, mostly because contradictory religious beliefs have led to so many wars and atrocities throughout the centuries. Therefore, it is with great sensitivity that I broach this topic and its potential relationship with physical healing. The mere mention of "spiritual healing" often polarizes a room—those with a strong spiritual practice will perk up immediately, while those without any spiritual beliefs or practices will abruptly shut down. My hope is that you will read this chapter somewhere in between, with an openness to accept other people's experiences while also knowing that some or all of it may not ring true for you.

In its simplest form, this chapter discusses the idea of physical healing due to one's connection to a deeper (or higher) energy, which some people personalize as "God," some call "the soul," and others generalize as a ubiquitous life force, calling it "energy," "chi," or "prana." For the sake of this chapter, I will refer to it as "spiritual energy," but if you are a person who cringes at the word "spiritual," you can just mentally replace the words "spiritual energy" with "deep, peaceful energy."

There are five aspects of spiritual energy that Radical Remission survivors and alternative healers describe frequently. After exploring them in depth, we will dive into a Radical Remission healing story about a young man with brain cancer who used spiritual energy for healing, and finally we'll conclude with some simple action steps you can take to start developing your own spiritual connection practice.

SPIRITUALITY AS AN EXPERIENCE

The Radical Remission survivors and alternative healers I study describe spiritual energy as something they feel simultaneously as both a physical sensation and an intense emotion. It is typically described as a feeling of warm, peaceful energy that flows downward, from head to toe, coating both the physical and emotional bodies with a blanket of deep peace and unconditional love. Many people assume that feeling spiritual energy requires you to have spiritual or religious beliefs. This is simply not true. This feeling of blissful, spiritual energy is not the result of a *belief* but rather a mental and/ or physical practice that produces an intense *experience* of spiritual energy.

For example, someone may experience spiritual energy to varying degrees after a good yoga class, a long run, a relaxing massage, or an afternoon nap. There are also spiritual practices designed specifically to elicit this experience, such as deep prayer, meditation, or chanting. As with most things in life, everyone responds to things differently. For some people, they may never feel a spiritual "buzz" after a yoga class, but feel it intensely at their weekly prayer circle.

Others may have difficulty feeling spiritual energy while meditating, yet feel it easily when they are walking in nature. According to the people I study, the method of connecting to this spiritual energy does not matter; it only matters that you *do* connect, daily if possible, in order to receive its healing benefits.

Sister Jayanti is an expert at introducing newcomers to the spiritual connection practice of meditation. Jayanti is a leader of the Brahma Kumaris World Spiritual Organization, a primarily women-led spiritual group dedicated to teaching nondenominational spirituality and meditation. She describes meditation as one way to have an experience of spiritual energy:

Where you're in deep communion, in deep conversation, or even in deep silence, but just in the presence of the divine—that's meditation. . . . So, in that state of union, what happens is you're drawing that light, that energy, not just into the soul but also from the soul, and the rays extend out into the body also. It's like the warmth of the sun. You can feel that energy, not just on a superficial level on your skin but you can feel your body absorbing that warmth and that energy within itself. . . . It actually is a process of healing. It actually helps the body heal. . . . The primary advice given to persons with a physical illness, therefore, is to practice meditation and to be mindful of every thought and action. These practices help to connect the person back to the divine energy source, which is the primary aspect of their being.

Radical Remission survivor Bridget Dinsmore also describes connecting to spiritual energy as being key to her healing. Bridget was diagnosed with uterine cancer and given five years to live, as long as she agreed to receive an immediate hysterectomy followed by intensive chemotherapy and radiation. However, she had just finished reading Louise Hay's book *Heal Your Body* and was inspired by the author's description of the body's ability to self-heal. Therefore, Bridget decided to postpone any medical treatment for a few months so she could try what she calls "spiritual healing," which, among other things, included practicing guided imagery and Reiki regularly in order to go inward. She describes her journey as follows:

> At first, I had no clue what spiritual healing was all about. Although I was brought up in a very strict religious faith [Catholicism], I hadn't been practicing it, so I was off on an adventure of my own. Little did I know that the spiritual healer was myself! I found that out after I had been diagnosed as cancer-free the following year, and most of my healing was just looking at and connecting with my inner self.

Even though Bridget had been raised in a particular faith, her exact spiritual beliefs did not matter as much as the spiritual practices she learned in order to experience that peaceful, spiritual energy on a daily basis. I find that many people today are disillusioned with weekly religious services that feel rote and outdated, yet they attend them out of obligation; meanwhile, experience-based activities such as yoga or running are gaining in popularity. Perhaps that is because having spiritual energy actually course through our bodies and minds nourishes us more than having spiritual beliefs that live only in our heads.

A THIRD TYPE OF LOVE

In other chapters, we have discussed the importance of feeling positive emotions, such as joy and love (chapter 6), and receiving love and support from others (chapter 7). However, both of these types of love relate to love on an individual level. For example, when it comes to positive emotions, we can focus on activities and thoughts that lead to our own individual selves feeling more positive and loving; or, when it comes to social support, we can focus on learning how to receive love from other individuals.

This chapter looks at a third type of love, what I call spiritual energy and what many of the people I study refer to as "unconditional, universal love." When they describe feeling this love, they say they lose a sense of separateness from all other things—they no longer feel like an individual but instead feel merged with everyone and everything. This feeling starts to flood their whole being when they engage in a spiritual practice; it comes from no particular source and is directed toward all things. They describe it as a deep, universal love that is available to us in every situation, but only if we actively tap into it. It is like having a healing river flowing under the ground at all times—the river is always there, but you have to take the time to stop, dig a hole, and drink the water if you want to receive its healing benefits.

One Radical Remission survivor who discovered this third type of love is "Henry." Henry was diagnosed at age seventy with both prostate and male breast cancer, but he turned down the recommended surgery and chemotherapy, and instead investigated other forms of healing. This led him to discover Tong Ren, a spiritual practice that is an offshoot of Traditional Chinese Medicine. Henry's teacher, a licensed acupuncturist named Tom Tam, introduced Henry to the idea that there is a universal, spiritual energy to which everyone can connect in order to help heal their physical ailments, such as cancer. Henry explains:

Tom has the idea that we have a larger cultural mind—he calls it a collective unconscious—and that the more we engage that [collective unconscious], or the more the [Tong Ren] practitioner is just sort of a conduit of that [collective unconscious], then that larger conscious mind has the power to heal, which is the same as almost every other culture that talks about healing.

Tong Ren was the practice Henry used to connect to this third type of love—the unconditional and universal type—in order to help heal his cancer. He never received any conventional medical treatment, and although he passed away at age eighty-three, he still amazed his doctors by living for thirteen years after his double diagnosis.

We live in a culture that prioritizes individualism above all else. We are taught to become individual citizens who live independent, separate lives from our neighbors. However, all the major spiritual traditions tell us the exact opposite, that we are all intimately and invisibly connected and that, in fact, we are all made of the same spiritual energy. If you have never had an experience of universal love, where the feeling that you are an individual slips away and you feel merged with and at peace with everything, then you probably have not yet had a full experience of this third kind of love, which many Radical Remission survivors describe as "the deepest love there is."

THE RELATIONSHIP BETWEEN PHYSICAL AND SPIRITUAL

One idea related to spiritual energy that comes up again and again in my research is the notion that humans are primarily spiritual beings having a temporary, physical experience in a body. When it comes to healing cancer, this idea becomes important when it influences someone's course of treatment. For example, if you believe we are only physical organisms, then you would only look for physical causes of cancer and physical treatments for it. But if you believe the spiritual energy *inside* physical bodies needs just as much care as the physical bodies, then you will look beyond just the physical.

Many of the people I study believe that the soul or spiritual energy aspect of humans is the most important aspect of ourselves, and if we forget to connect to that aspect on a regular basis, the body will eventually get run-down or sick. One alternative healer who believes this is a man named Swami Brahmdev, founder of a yoga and meditation ashram in northern India. Brahmdev believes that deepening your connection to the spiritual energy within each of us should be the first step in any physical healing process. He explains this in his rhythmic voice:

> *This box [points to his body] is made for the divine. So, [the] divine is living inside of everyone. . . . And if you think that now you are suffering with [an illness], at least now become aware of that and awaken that divinity, involve that divinity, and tell that divine force to help you, to protect you, to save you, to cure you—and* involve *the divinity. Grow your faith in the divine in you. This [points to his body] is not* your *home; this is not* your *box. This box belongs to the divine. . . . And now this home is in danger [i.e., illness has occurred], so at least now tell the owner of the home, "Please, teach me. I am not able to keep you good with me, so please come out. Help me."*

In other words, Swami Brahmdev views the human body as a container for divine energy, similar to how many religions view the body as a container for the soul. According to him, reestablishing and strengthening one's connection to this divine energy inside each of us is the best way to care for this "box" that is the physical body, especially when it becomes ill. Not all the people I interview feel as strongly as Brahmdev does about the primacy of the spirit over the physical body; however, almost all of them believe that spiritual energy is an important aspect of who we are as human beings and connecting to it regularly can significantly help the physical body heal.

THE IMPORTANCE OF REGULAR PRACTICE

Most people read accounts of spiritual healing in which a person is flooded with spiritual energy, merges with the "oneness," and heals shortly thereafter, and they think to themselves, *That may have happened, but it will never happen to me.* I used to be one of those people, because I did not know I could slowly develop a practice that allowed me to feel more palpably the sensation of spiritual energy coursing through my body. In many of the spiritual healing stories we read, people are flooded with this spiritual energy instantly and inexplicably, without much effort on their part.

However, one thing I have learned from Radical Remission survivors is that, while some may be lucky enough to experience an instant flood of spiritual energy, most of us have to work up to it slowly with regular, committed practice. The analogy I like to use is weight lifting. You cannot walk into a gym having not lifted a weight in five years (or more!) and expect suddenly to bench-press two hundred pounds. Similarly, you cannot sit on a meditation cushion having never meditated and expect to have spiritual energy instantly inundate your entire being. Rather, just like the weight lifter, you need to start small and build up your ability with regular—ideally daily—practice. Furthermore, just like weight lifting, if you take a month off from your practice, you cannot necessarily jump back in where you left off; instead, you may have to start back at the beginning.

Sister Jayanti commented on how most people these days do not have a regular spiritual practice because it is not considered as important in our culture as "getting things done":

What's happened in recent times is that instead of human "beings," we've become human "doings," and so we just get caught up in the doing, the doing, the action. The process of spirituality is to be able to look inside and see what's going on within *the soul and to come back to that state of being in which I can be at peace with myself. . . . So that when I'm aware of who I am in my original state of being, I am peaceful. And when I forget who I am, I lose that peace and I lose contact with myself.*

In other words, Jayanti believes that a healthy human is one who regularly connects the action-oriented body to the peace-oriented soul. I know that when I am meditating regularly, peaceful, spiritual energy fills my body quickly and stays with me for most of my day. However, when I meditate sporadically—usually because I am "too busy" with life—that connection is very difficult to make and I feel only a small amount of that peaceful energy trickling through my body. According to Jayanti and many of the other people I interview, the consequences of not connecting regularly to spiritual energy are not to be taken lightly: at first, you may start to feel a general lack of peace in your life, but eventually physical illness can develop, because the body is not "recharging its batteries" (i.e., connecting to spiritual energy) on a regular basis like it should. Therefore, as with so many other things in this world, the take-home message is simple: practice, practice, practice.

THE IMPORTANCE OF STOPPING THE MIND

The fifth aspect of deepening spirituality is the idea that, regardless of which spiritual practice you choose—prayer, meditation, running, yoga, etc.—the first step of connecting to spiritual energy is quieting your mind. The two seem to be mutually exclusive: spiritual energy cannot start to flow through your body before the thoughts in your mind have stopped. This is by far one of the biggest barriers to regular spiritual practice, as so many of us today have trouble shutting off our thoughts, especially given the overwhelming amount of information we are bombarded with each day. The mere fact that 48 percent of Americans struggle with occasional insomnia and 40 million people in the United States also suffer from anxiety tells us that we are indeed having trouble turning off our minds.[1]

Each spiritual practice has its own set of tricks for shutting off the thinking mind. In most meditation practices, for example, you do not try to quiet the mind at all but rather step back and simply observe your racing thoughts. By distancing yourself from your thoughts in this way, the thoughts slowly calm down and eventually dissipate. Other tricks for stopping one's thoughts include focusing on something else, such as a repeated prayer, a mantra, an image, or your breath. Many people find that exercising is another great way to clear the mind before engaging in a spiritual practice such as prayer or meditation. Again, it is not the method of stopping your thoughts that matters, only that you *do* find a way to silence your racing mind, so the true experience of spiritual energy can begin.

"Rita" is a researcher by occupation, so she is constantly in her thinking mind. When Rita was diagnosed with breast cancer, she first treated it with conventional medicine, but unfortunately it recurred a few years later. She was very angry with God when she first found out about her recurrence; however, this anger actually helped her get out of her thinking mind:

> *I walked out to the street and I said, "God, if you are who you say you are, then you do it." You know? I was pissed. I said, "You heal me or kill me. Just do it fast." I'm a researcher by nature, but I said, "I'm not doing another thing. I'm not talking to anybody else. No more libraries, no more books—nothing. You do it."* . . . *And in a week and a half, things started to change.*

Later that week, a set of strange coincidences led Rita to try a new energy-healing treatment and to intensify her meditation practice. She also chose not to jump back into conventional medicine right away. After a month of meditating and receiving the energy-healing treatment, her breast tumor was no longer palpable to the touch. Her healing journey continued, and although she chose never to return to conventional doctors, and therefore has never verified that her cancer has indeed gone away, she is currently—more than twenty-four years later—loving life and enjoying excellent health. For Rita, deepening her spiritual practice required her first to turn off her thinking, researching mind. The Radical Remission survivors and alternative healers I study all say that this step is absolutely essential if we want to be able to access the spiritual energy inside all of us.

SPIRITUALITY RESEARCH

We will talk at the end of this chapter about some ways in which you can start to connect to spiritual energy, but first I would like to let you know about some of the recent research that has been conducted on this topic. Thanks to the relatively new inventions of fMRI (functional magnetic resonance imaging), EEG (electroencephalography), and blood plasma spinners, researchers are now able to study the effects that spiritual connection practices have on the brain and the body—and the results so far have been very intriguing.

For example, researchers have found that practicing meditation produces high levels of melatonin in the body.[2] Melatonin is a healthy and necessary hormone that helps us sleep. A good night's sleep is vital to our health, because it is the only time when our immune systems can spend hours repairing cells and cleaning out the body.[3] Interestingly, melatonin has been found to be dangerously low in many cancer patients.[4] Therefore, this study could explain how a spiritual practice such as meditation might help the body fight cancer.

In another study, researchers found that meditating for just thirty minutes a day for eight weeks decreases the density of your brain areas associated with anxiety and stress and increases your brain matter density in the areas associated with empathy and memory.[5] This study is important for cancer patients because countless studies have shown that decreasing stress boosts your immune system.[6] So, because meditation is a proven stress reliever, it is therefore also an immune booster.

Other studies have looked directly at meditation's effects on the immune system. One such study showed that the more you meditate, the more virus antibodies you produce.[7] This is an important finding for cancer patients because more cancers are being linked to viruses (e.g., HPV has been linked to cervical cancer). In another study on the immune system, meditation was shown to significantly increase telomerase activity in immune system cells.[8] Telomerase is commonly known as the antiaging enzyme because it allows cells to live longer. So, in this study, meditation allowed people's immune system cells to live longer, which is a good thing when the body is trying to fight cancer.

Finally, epigenetics is a new and exciting field of science that studies how human behavior can affect gene expression. In a nutshell, epigenetics has shown that, while we may not be able to change which genes we inherit from our parents, we can—through our behavior—change whether or not those genes are turned on or off (i.e., expressed or not expressed). Keep in mind that a faulty gene you have inherited can only hurt you if it is turned on. In terms of spiritual practice, one recent study showed that beginner meditators significantly changed their gene expression in a health-promoting way after just eight weeks of regular meditation practice.[9] In other words, a spiritual practice such as meditation can actually turn healthy genes on and unhealthy genes off. This is an incredible discovery for cancer patients, because it means they do not need to be so fearful if they are carriers of cancer genes (i.e., oncogenes), such as the BRCA mutation in breast cancer patients. Instead, cancer patients who have these oncogenes can focus on certain behaviors—diet, spiritual practice, exercise, etc.—that have the potential to turn those genes off.

Most of the convincing research on spiritual practice so far has been done on meditation, yoga, and tai chi, but not on prayer. This is because it is very difficult to measure the strength or quality of one's prayers. Meditation studies are easier to design, because you can take a group of people and lead them through concrete steps that teach them how to meditate. This does not mean that meditation is the best spiritual practice there is; it just means it is one of the easier spiritual practices to measure. I hope, in years to come, researchers will figure out better ways to measure the effects prayer has on the physical body. Until then, the spate of well-designed studies on meditation, yoga, and tai chi have shown conclusively that these spiritual practices improve the health of the body (e.g., improved circulation, better sleep, stronger immune system) and the mind (e.g., less stress, more empathy).

I WOULD NOW like to share with you the healing story of Matthew, a young man who was diagnosed with terminal brain cancer at the tender age of twenty-seven, tried everything Western medicine had to offer, and yet was sent home on hospice care. With nothing left to lose, he embarked on an unexpected journey of daily spiritual practice that led him to places he never could have imagined.

—∾ Matthew's Story ∾—

In 2002, Matthew had recently graduated from college and invested what little savings he had in a small piece of land in the Colorado mountains, near his brother. Despite the tranquil location, he was very busy commuting between two jobs—one as a maintainer of camping huts in the Rocky Mountain hiking system and the other as a high school basketball coach. He recalls the demands of his life at that time:

> *Every morning at five A.M. I would drive almost an hour to work. I would work all day, and then I would drive another hour, where I was coaching a high school basketball team. And then after practice I would drive another hour back [home]. . . . So, it was a lot of time on the road. I was just pushing myself too much, I think, too much beyond my limits.*

Matthew appreciated the fact that his job allowed him to exercise and be out in nature every day, but the job was also the most physically demanding he had ever had. Every day he would have to walk many miles in high altitudes carrying heavy supplies, such as firewood, to the camping huts. On top of that, his daily driving schedule left him little time for a social life or sleep. He was no longer living with friends as he had during college, he was still healing from a recent romantic breakup, and he remembers feeling a bit depressed in general.

It was during this time that Matthew's headaches began. One day around ten in the morning he got a fairly strong headache, but it passed after a few hours, so he thought nothing of it. The same thing happened the next morning—an unusually strong headache struck around ten, which faded after a few hours. This went on for a few days, getting worse and lasting longer with each day. He saw a massage therapist and a chiropractor, but both provided only temporary relief. A local doctor diagnosed him with migraines, but even heavy-duty painkillers did not help with the pain. After two weeks, the pain was lasting around the clock and was so severe that it was making Matthew vomit. Unfortunately, because he had invested all his money in buying his piece of land, he did not have any health insurance at that time, but his boss gave him some sound advice:

> [My boss] said, "Listen. Why don't you go to the hospital and get an MRI? . . . If you have to pay ten dollars a year for the rest of your life to pay for it, at least go and count out the very worst."

Matthew was able to get in for the last MRI of the day at a nearby hospital, and he remembers writhing in pain on the waiting room couch. Finally, the results came in:

> The doctor told me, "There's something in your head. We don't know what it is yet, but it has to be dealt with immediately. Tonight. We don't have the facilities at our hospital to do this kind of surgery, but you have to go get this removed right now or—or you're going to put your life at risk."

Tears came to Matthew's eyes as he recalled this moment during our interview. Clearly, receiving that shocking news was still an incredibly powerful memory for him, even years later. After the MRI, and while still in severe pain, he broke the news to his parents back on the East Coast, his best friend, and his brother who lived an hour away. His mother immediately hopped on an airplane, and his brother jumped into a car and drove an hour to pick up Matthew, and then drove them eight additional hours to a bigger hospital in Denver.

The doctors in Denver ran a second MRI to verify the location of Matthew's tumor, and their worst fears were confirmed. It was located in the very center of his brain, which meant it was inoperable. They explained that his headaches were being caused by a severe backup of cerebral-spinal fluid, which the tumor was preventing from flowing as it should. The doctors planned to drill a hole into Matthew's brain and insert an emergency shunt, which would divert the fluid around the tumor, thereby relieving the pressure. If they did not operate, the pressure of the fluid would increase over the next few days until the vessels in his head burst, killing him. In other words, this surgery was by no means optional. With the help of social workers at the hospital, Matthew immediately signed up for his state's emergency health insurance plan for people with life-threatening conditions.

By the time he was wheeled into surgery twenty-four hours later, he was already surrounded by his mother, brother, and friends. Tears of gratitude choked Matthew's voice during our interview as he described this scene:

My brother stayed up there with me, and then a dear friend from the area came too. And my mom flew cross-country. And two of my friends—brothers, really—who were my roommates in college and are lifetime friends, they just dropped everything they were doing and came to be with me. And this was so powerful. . . . It was the first time in my life that I realized how many people really, really *loved me. When it comes down to it—and I believe this very much—what healed me was the power of love. And that comes from many facets. One of those was very much my family and my friends.*

The surgery itself was incredibly risky, but luckily the doctors operated skillfully and Matthew came out of it with no complications and no further headaches. He still had a very large tumor in the center of his brain, though. During the surgery, the doctors were able to snip off a piece of the tumor and confirm that it was "inoperable stage 4 glioblastoma," the most aggressive form of brain cancer found in humans.

A few days later, Matthew underwent a second surgery in which his temporary, external shunt was converted to a permanent, internal shunt. Before he was discharged, the doctor called him in to discuss his treatment plan and explained that conventional medicine did not understand this type of cancer very well. He went on to say that the best-case scenario would be if chemotherapy and radiation were to simply slow the tumor's growth, thereby giving Matthew more months to live:

The doctor said, "I suggest that you go be near your family where you can have that support. I would give you, honestly, a 1 or 2 percent chance of being as good as you are now or any better in twelve to sixteen weeks." . . . He was fully honest, and God bless him. He saved my life [by inserting the shunt], and I thank him endlessly for that. But what I came to find out over the next couple of years is that he did everything he could, but he stopped

where he didn't know what to do—and that's where something
bigger helped me.

Later that night, the doctor's sobering news was finally sinking
in. And then, ever so slowly, a new feeling began to bubble up in
Matthew: defiance.

Excuse my language, but I wanted to say to my doctor, "You
know what? Fuck you. I'm not ready to die! And if you give me
a 1 or 2 percent chance, that's fine. I'll do it! That's me. I'm
gonna be that 1 or 2 percent chance, and I'm gonna beat this,
and I don't care if nobody else has. You can be wrong." I wish so
much that more people would take that attitude and have faith
in themselves. If anything else, that could be one of the biggest,
biggest healers in the world—if people just believed and had
some hope.

Matthew followed his doctor's advice and moved back to the
East Coast where he could be closer to his family and friends while
undergoing the recommended radiation and chemotherapy. As soon
as he was physically able after recovering from the surgery, he began
daily gamma-knife radiation treatments to his brain:

They'd shoot these three different lasers into my brain, from three
different angles, and it would burn where they all joined in the
center. And so basically what they were trying to do was burn
the tumor out of there, to extract it without being intrusive—
well, physically intrusive, I should say. [laughs] That's a lot of
radiation and it's very powerful. If I were to go through this
again, I'm not sure if I would do it.

At the same time, advice was pouring in from friends and family about all the things he should be doing for his health. Willing to try anything that might help, Matthew tried acupuncture, cranial-sacral work, and energy healing—all of which were firsts. His doctors also wanted to treat his cancer with chemotherapy at the same time they were giving him the gamma-knife radiation. However, Matthew was hesitant because his doctors had told him that only 30 percent or less of the chemotherapy would ever reach his tumor due to the body's inherent blood–brain barrier. The other 70 percent would go to the rest of his body, causing unnecessary and painful side effects. On top of that, there was only a 30 percent chance that any of the chemotherapy drugs would actually be able to shrink his tumor. In fact, the research was so ambiguous that Matthew was told *he* could pick which chemotherapy he wanted to try. Nevertheless, the doctors encouraged the chemotherapy because it was their only additional strategy. Matthew eventually agreed to try one that he could take in pill form:

> *I tell you, after two weeks of it, I threw [the chemotherapy] in the trash! It was miserable. I don't know if what I was feeling were the side effects of the radiation or the chemotherapy or the combination thereof, but it had come to a point where anything I put into my mouth tasted like wet cardboard. I could eat a spoonful of salt and not even know it was salt. . . . I said, "If I'm not going to make it through this, I'd like to make it as myself. I don't want to be this thing that doesn't enjoy any food, that can't recognize people."*

Soon afterward, Matthew reached the maximum amount of radiation allowable for humans. Unfortunately, his tumor was still growing. However, the rate at which it was growing had slowed somewhat. His doctors told him there was nothing else they could offer him, except to monitor him with scans. He left the hospital believing the horrible side effects of the radiation had been worth it, because at least he had bought some time. The rest was up to him, and whatever complementary treatments he was willing to try.

One of Matthew's friends knew of a shaman in Peru who led small groups of people on "healing journeys" and had apparently had some remarkable successes. Therefore, when Matthew's friend offered to accompany him to see this shaman, he was open to trying it. However, by this point, his medical procedures had sent him into significant debt, and he could not afford the cost of the trip. When his friends and family learned of this, they immediately organized a fund-raiser for him. Matthew was deeply moved by this act of kindness, and also by something special that happened at the fund-raiser:

> A stranger was walking down the street and saw something happening, so she came in and asked what was going on. [My friends] explained to her, and she said, "Well, I don't have much, but I'll give you everything I have in my pocket, and I pray it can do some good." And this was a total, complete stranger coming in off the street and giving charity—not just the charity of money, but a charity that's so much more powerful: the charity of love. You know? Just totally unbiased, unconditional love. To help another human like that was really, really powerful for me.

After this fund-raiser, Matthew was able to buy the ticket to Peru and was scheduled to leave in a few weeks. During that time, the woman who was going to accompany him received a phone call from one of her friends who was also going on the trip. The friend said she had had a strong intuition: "Matthew doesn't need to come to Peru with us. He needs to go see John of God in Brazil." When Matthew heard this message, he was confused. Who was John of God? He decided to do some online research. He had already researched numerous other healers in his search for potential treatments, and a lot of them "just seemed bogus" to him. However, he was intrigued by the fact that this healer, João Teixeira de Faria (nicknamed John of God by his patients), did not charge for his healing work:

> *One thing that caught me about this man was that it was a free clinic. He did it for* free. . . . *First, I didn't have a lot of money to go pay thousands of dollars to try something, but also, just the idea that someone is not healing for money. . . . That sort of convinced me that this man really wants to heal people.*

While the free aspect appealed to Matthew, the rest of João's healing work sounded incredibly strange. Apparently, this man had the ability to leave his body and go into a trance, thereby allowing the spirit of a higher being to enter his body and perform energetic healing work. Although it sounded crazy, Matthew was nevertheless inspired by the large number of cancer patients who had apparently been healed by this man. He was intrigued enough that he looked into changing his ticket from Peru to Brazil, but it turned out that his ticket was neither refundable nor changeable. So, Matthew accepted that he would go to Peru as planned and perhaps visit John of God at a later date.

Two weeks before he was to leave for Peru, Matthew was spending some time with friends, knowing full well that this might be the last time he saw them. As strong as his will to live was, his prognosis was weighing heavily on him during those days. One morning, the friends' next-door neighbor—a woman he had never met but who had heard about Matthew's situation—called to tell him that John of God had healed her breast cancer. This was the second time Matthew was hearing about John of God from a complete stranger, and he remembers being shaken by the coincidence. She invited him over so she could share her story, and she also showed him a video of John of God sending healing energy to someone.

The neighbor's story and video only piqued Matthew's desire to visit John of God, but he told her he couldn't because of the nonrefundable Peru tickets. He thanked her for her time and assured her that he would visit John of God as soon as he could afford it. Matthew describes her response:

> What she said to me was a wonderful piece of love. . . . She said, "If you want to go, I'll buy you a ticket right now. And I will set you up there. And you pay me back as soon as you can. If your heart tells you to do this for your healing, I do not want money to be the ridiculous thing that holds you back." So, I walked home with a ticket to the middle of central Brazil with only three weeks to prepare! It was crazy how all this happened. And sure enough, I paid her back. She was the first person I paid back, as fast as I could. These are the little things that are all tied in with that power of love that I believe is so powerful in healing.

In the weeks that followed, Matthew continued to meet strangers who had either just been to see John of God or whose friend had just been there, all with positive things to say. On the plane to Brazil, the man seated next to him was also on his way to see John of God. To Matthew, all these things seemed to be saying, "Yes. You're finally hearing me. You're finally listening." That is how, in November of 2003, he found himself alone, in a basic hotel room, in the middle of a rural Brazilian town named Abadiânia, with a stage 4 brain tumor, preparing to see a healer named John of God.

AT AROUND TWO in the morning, Matthew woke up and noticed that his bathroom light was on. Exhausted, he shut his eyes and rolled over, trying to ignore it. The light was keeping him from falling back asleep, though, so he eventually got up to turn it off. Matthew describes what happened next:

I kind of open my eyes and I look over, and I see that it's not really the bathroom light. There's something in there moving— there's someone in there. And then there was a woman walking out of there, and she was just shrouded in light. I can't see her face exactly, but she was just this beautiful, beautiful light. I can't describe the color, but it was like . . . the perfect light. She was walking slowly over to me, and she didn't say anything, but she held out her hand. And then she was right beside me, and she reached out her hand, and she put it on my head.

And in that instant, from my head down slowly, it trickled like it was paint oozing down my body, inside and out, like every nerve in my body, every piece of my body could feel it, and it just flooded me. I just kind of closed my eyes and let it take me over. And it was just this feeling of—I think it was the feeling of perfection. Of pure, pure love. Of unhaltered charity, of bliss, of ecstasy, of perfection. And it flooded me for several seconds, and I held on to it. And then I opened my eyes and it [the feeling and the woman] was gone.

And then I realize that I am sitting there, and I'm wide awake on my bed, and I realize very much that I didn't dream this. This just happened and it was so real. I mean I could still feel it tingling in my body. This was the most powerful thing I've ever felt in my life. And maybe I didn't know it yet, but that was love. That's what love is. And that's what God is.

Nothing like this had ever happened to Matthew before. He had not been raised with religion, and he had never attended church. Before this experience, he did not believe in any particular religion. As he describes it, the closest thing he had to a feeling of God was the way he felt when he was in nature, among the trees and sunlight. In fact, he had always been turned *off* by religion due to its many historical wars and scandals. Despite all of this, the experience he had with the "spirit" in his bathroom moved him to his core and awakened something in him that he now calls faith:

> *I think faith is something every human being has inside, but sometimes we never find it, sometimes it never wakes up— because of our own fault, no one else's. Sometimes we ignore it. But I very much believe that we all have faith. And mine awoke that first night, and as my experiences in Abadiânia continued, that faith just grew stronger and stronger, and my decision to live, and not to die, just grew stronger and stronger with it.*

THE NEXT MORNING, Matthew waited in line with approximately five hundred other people in order to see John of God one on one for about ten seconds, thereby receiving a burst of his high-powered energy. As instructed, they had all put on white clothes (which, they were told, allowed the "spirits" to read their energy field more quickly) and began inching forward in line, slowly moving through two meditation rooms before finally seeing John of God. When Matthew reached the front of the line and told John of God (via a translator) that he wanted his brain cancer healed, John of God looked at him intensely for a moment—simultaneously reading Matthew's energy field and giving him a burst of high-powered energy—and then instructed him (via the translator) to do two things: first, start taking energetically infused passionflower herbs every day, and second, meditate daily in the main meditation room (the same room in which John of God sits and sees patients).

On the three days of each week that John of God sees patients, about a hundred people are invited to sit and meditate in the same room where he sits. This is called the "current room," because of the strong current of energy that is supposedly present in the room. Some people, like Matthew, are instructed by John of God to sit in the room because they need healing, while others are healthy volunteers who have been asked by John of God to sit in the room to help "hold" the strong energy in the room. Following John of God's recommendations, Matthew began meditating in the current room during the three days a week John of God sees patients, and he also began taking the passionflower herbs. His plan was to stay at the healing center for about a month, and he quickly fell into the routine of meditating with John of God by day and resting and eating at the small hotel by night. The hotels in Abadiânia, which are really more like hostels, are very inexpensive and include three home-cooked meals a day. Matthew was lucky that his family and friends were willing to support the minor cost of the hotel; the healing from John of God was, however, completely free.

During one of his first days there, while Matthew was meditating in the current room with his eyes closed (as instructed), the person next to him gently picked up Matthew's hand, lifted it up to Matthew's head, and rested it there. Confused, Matthew kept his eyes closed, left his hand on his head for a few seconds, and then slowly lowered it back down to his lap. Immediately, the stranger picked up Matthew's hand again and placed it on top of Matthew's head, this time patting it. Matthew understood the silent message that he was to keep his hand on his head.

Then something amazing happened. After a few moments, he

began to feel that same, blissful sensation of oozing light traveling from his hand down his body, just as it had his first night at the hotel. After a few minutes of experiencing this bliss, the stranger gently removed Matthew's hand from his head and rested it again in Matthew's lap. Matthew just sat there in awe of what had transpired. At the end of the meditation session a few hours later, he finally opened his eyes and turned to the stranger in gratitude:

> *I looked over at this total stranger—who has become a very, very dear friend since then—and I said, "Thank you!" And he said, "For what?" And I said, "For doing this!" and I put my hand on my head. Here I am thinking,* How does this guy know I've got a brain tumor? How does he have any idea of this?! *And he said, "Oh, that wasn't me. Spirit told me to do that."*

Most people see John of God for only one to two weeks, but very occasionally John of God will recommend that a person stay in Abadiânia long-term until he or she is fully healed. Matthew was one of those people, and because of the amazing things he had experienced in just his first week, he didn't mind staying on. Besides, it's not like he had any other healing options back home. He did miss his family and friends dearly at times, but he also felt that he was making progress at John of God's, whereas back home his only option would be hospice care. His friends and family graciously continued to support the small cost of his hotel, even if some of them were still skeptical of this alternative mode of healing.

After about a month of taking the herbs every day and meditating in the current room for six hours a day, three days a week, John of God instructed Matthew to get his first "energetic surgery." This is not a physical surgery, but rather a fifteen- to thirty-minute meditation in a room with others who are also receiving an energetic surgery. Matthew explains that the spirits who work through John of God apparently use this surgery time to adjust a person's energy field. They are called surgeries because the spirits apparently cut, unblock, and/or repair your energetic meridians, just as a Western surgeon might cut, unblock, and/or repair your arteries. These energetic surgeries are noninvasive, painless, and tend to make the person feel incredibly sleepy afterward. For example, it is not uncommon for a person to sleep sixteen to twenty-four hours after receiving one of them. Matthew enjoyed the calming, sleep-inducing experience of his first energetic surgery, and then—as instructed—he returned to his routine of meditating in the current room three days a week and taking the herbs every day.

In their brief interactions, John of God never called Matthew's condition "cancer." Instead, he simply said (via a translator), "Something very powerful is in your head." Also, a few times while meditating in the current room with his eyes closed, Matthew sensed John of God approaching him. John of God would then place his hand on Matthew's head, and that feeling of blissful light would instantly start pouring through him again.

After three months like this at John of God's center, Matthew's visitor visa had run out, so he returned to the United States to see his family and renew his visa. He did this for the rest of that year, spending three months at a time in Abadiânia and returning to the United States only to renew his visa. His family happily paid for his plane tickets home, and when they saw how much better he looked, they didn't hesitate to pay for his return flights to Brazil or to keep paying for the inexpensive hotel. When I asked Matthew why he chose to stay at John of God's for so long, he replied:

I said, "If I'm gonna do this, I'm gonna do it." I didn't know
it then, but now I would call that faith. You've got to believe

in something. And you can't just go into something halfway. I
believe you just do it. And you don't need to shotgun everything
and try this and that and that. Just choose what you believe in. I
mean, I might believe in spirit and in the power of God now. But
"Joshua" might believe in chemotherapy 100 percent, with all of
his heart. And that might work for him. But that might not do a
thing for me. There is a power in [believing in your treatment],
and I don't know where one leaves off [belief versus treatment],
but the power of faith and what we can do for ourselves is so
much bigger than I think most of us understand.

Meanwhile, Matthew's doctors wanted him to come in for another MRI, but Matthew kept postponing it. He was not only afraid that his tumor might still be growing but also afraid that he would be letting down his friends and family. After all, they had raised the money to allow him to try other treatments. Even though he felt strongly that something powerful was happening at John of God's center, he did not want a possible "bad" MRI to shake his newly found faith. So, for that first year, he ignored his doctors' requests.

Then one day, after he'd been at John of God's for about a year, Matthew was home in the United States visiting his family when he suddenly felt ready to get an MRI. He told only his mother, and they secretly went without telling anyone else. John of God had not yet told him that he was officially "healed," which John of God will say to people who have been seeing him for a long time. Nevertheless, Matthew was ready to see if any improvement could be detected by conventional technology. After the MRI, a doctor finally came to give him the news:

A wonderful radiologist came and talked to us. He said, "I have
great news!" At this point, I thought that maybe the tumor was

gone, but I didn't want to have too much hope. He said, "It looks like from the pictures and all the angles that we've taken that your tumor is still there, but it has shrunk considerably."

After he heard this news, Matthew's faith "shot up by a hundred points." What was equally amazing to him, though, was how the news boosted the faith of his family and friends. One of his dearest friends had grown up in a family of doctors. In her world, if something went wrong with your body, you went to the doctor to have it "fixed." She never believed that John of God would actually help Matthew, but she had still been supportive of him as a friend. After Matthew told her the news, she called him in tears and said, "You get your ass back there as fast as you can, and you keep going with what you're doing!" The responses he received from all his friends and family that day were, as he describes, "amazing." Boosted by this wave of support, he returned to Abadiânia as soon as he could, and once again meditated in the current room three days a week. He believes that much of his healing resulted from that time in meditation:

I think that so much of what I could do to help in my healing was done in the current room, which seemed to me to be as strong as any surgery I could imagine. One of the organizers said one day, "Tell everybody that you know 'I forgive you.'" . . . Not just to say it, but to mean it." . . . It just seemed like something so good to do, to get rid of any negative energy that you hold in yourself or that might be between you and other people. Especially the people that you really disliked in the past, to find a way to say, "I'm really sorry. And I love you. I want the best for you." It doesn't mean you have to go hang out with them, but there's no reason to hang on to that negative energy. It's just such a waste for both people involved.

During this time, Matthew met a Brazilian woman who was also at John of God's center. She was not there for physical healing, but rather emotional healing. She was grieving the death of her brother, who had recently passed away from cancer, and the death of her father, who had passed away many years ago from the exact same brain cancer Matthew had. Given her past, it seems strangely coincidental that she would fall in love with someone who had the same cancer that had claimed her father's life. Nevertheless, fate often has a sense of irony, and she and Matthew fell in love instantly. As Matthew describes, their souls were "immediately drawn to one another."

Meanwhile, he continued to trust that his healing was progressing. Once, when John of God told him to have another energetic surgery, Matthew volunteered to have a physical surgery instead—one of those inexplicable, anesthesia-free surgeries he had seen on his friends' neighbor's video. He was at a point where he wanted to experience "absolutely everything" John of God had to offer, which is why he volunteered. John of God allows people to volunteer to undergo a physical surgery instead of an energetic one if they feel they need some sort of proof that something is being done to their bodies, even though he has said repeatedly that the energetic surgeries are just as effective as the physical ones. So, out of the fifty or so people who were told to have energetic surgeries that day, Matthew and two others requested a physical surgery:

> It came to my turn, and [John of God] stepped in front of me and said, "No. You do not need a physical surgery. What you need is spiritual work, and I want you to go back in that room and sit down right now, and I don't want you to come back here again." And so I got the message very, very clearly! [laughs]

More and more months went by with Matthew spending three days a week meditating in the current room, taking the herbs every day, and occasionally receiving energetic surgeries when instructed to by John of God. He spent the rest of his time getting to know the lovely Brazilian woman who had captured his heart from the moment he saw her, and after a year of courtship, they decided to get married in a small ceremony in Brazil.

———

ONE DAY, MATTHEW was sitting in the current room, meditating as usual. It had been almost two years to the day since he had first arrived at John of God's center, and it was also one day after his birthday. He was feeling happy and peaceful about his healing, his new marriage, and his life in Brazil. At the end of a long day of meditating, John of God was getting ready to lead the closing prayer. Before this happened, though, he approached Matthew and put his hand on Matthew's head, just as he had done several other times during Matthew's two years there. Once again, that wonderful feeling of blissful light poured through Matthew's body from John of God's hand. Then, however, something new happened:

[John of God] reached down and took my hand and he stood me up. [laughs] And he walked me up to the front of the room and turned me around. And he told the translator, "Now, I want you to turn around and face this room." Then he said, "Now I want you to tell everybody in this room exactly what you came here with two years ago and exactly what you have no more." [begins to cry]

It was the best day of my life! Then and there, I knew that the cancer was gone. And he went on to tell me, "I want you to go as soon as possible to a hospital and see a doctor and have an MRI.

And I want you to come back here with the proof that this tumor
is gone, because this will be something that will be very powerful
for many people in the future." And so I did, and I went, and
I had the MRI—and there was no more brain tumor in there!
[crying] It was my miracle.

After the good news had sunk in, Matthew and his wife decided
to stay in Abadiânia for a while. She had a good job that she was
not ready to leave, and Matthew was happy to spend more time
at John of God's center. He began volunteering at the center and
helped to organize the long lines of people each day. Other days he
would meditate in the current room to help "hold" the energy.

One day when he was volunteering, John of God passed by
Matthew and said, "I am [the spirit] known as José. I healed you."
Another day, John of God appeared to be channeling the spirit of
St. Ignatius, due to his distinct mannerisms, and said to Matthew,
"I healed you." (Note: John of God reportedly channels more than
thirty different spirits, also called "entities," which change depending on the needs of the particular patient.) When I asked Matthew
how he felt about the fact that two different spirits were claiming
credit for his healing, he replied:

What I understand is they all healed me. There is a spirit [at
John of God's center] named José that is oddly enough called "The
Spirit of Love." And so, again, that lends to the idea of the power
of love, and I think that love is very much what healed me in
many senses. I think that all the spirits work together. This is love.
This is God. They're all one—just as we're all part of the same
life. . . . I've always sort of understood the entities as the fingers of
God, doing the work of God.

In the end, Matthew spent a total of four years at John of God's center in Abadiânia, the first two of which were focused on his healing and the second two of which were spent volunteering and helping others in their healing process. At present, he and his wife split their time between the United States and Brazil and are expecting their second child, and Matthew continues to enjoy excellent health. His U.S. doctors remain completely baffled by his MRI, which shows no evidence of a brain tumor.

––––––––

WHEN I FIRST interviewed Matthew and heard his incredible healing story, I had to take an hour-long walk afterward just to digest it all, even though I had spent four weeks at John of God's center during my research trip and was therefore already familiar with the healing that occurs there. There is just something so moving about his story that it takes my breath away every time I hear it. Whether or not you agree with the choices he made, the fact remains that a young man who once had a fatal brain tumor is now cancer-free—and that is a beautiful thing.

So many things make Matthew's story powerful, not the least of which is the healer named John of God. As soon as I began announcing my dissertation research, numerous people insisted I visit his center in Brazil. After a bit of research, I found that hundreds of cancer patients had apparently healed there, so I decided to add it to my itinerary.

Before arriving, I read as many books as I could on the subject, one of the best being *John of God: The Brazilian Healer Who's Touched the Lives of Millions* by Heather Cumming and Karen Leffler. During my trip, my two stops before Brazil were Zambia and Zimbabwe, where alternative healers also believe in channeling higher spirits in order to transmit healing energy. So, by the time I arrived in Brazil, the idea of someone going into a trance in order to heal was not so foreign to me.

What I was not expecting was the palpable, calming energy field that seems to surround John of God's center—there really is no other way to describe it. For me and everyone else I met there, we were all able to meditate much faster and more deeply in that healing center as compared to back at home. Of course, this could simply be the placebo effect; in other words, our sheer belief that something powerful happens at John of God's center could have caused us to have a deeper meditation experience. Or a quicker and deeper meditation experience could be what happens whenever hundreds of people gather in one place to meditate. Regardless of its cause, we all found the "force field," as we jokingly called it, incredibly calming, sleep inducing, and healing.

I also was not expecting the surge of powerful energy I felt after seeing John of God in person. (In anthropological research, it is sometimes necessary to participate in the rituals one is studying in order to understand them more fully, and this principle certainly applied at John of God's center.) I later received an energetic surgery for my minor digestive complaint, and afterward I slept inexplicably for eighteen hours, which is something I have never done before. Finally, although it was minor, my lifelong digestive complaint resolved almost completely during my four weeks at the center, and it has not returned since.

Much more could be said about my time spent there, but in short I will say that the man called John of God seems to be able to transmit a very powerful surge of energy, which most people, myself included, experience as non-harmful, deeply relaxing, and physically and emotionally beneficial. Whether higher spirits are involved or not, I cannot say, but the exact mechanisms of the healing seem less important to me than the outcome.

Action Steps

If you are wondering whether you have to move to Brazil for two years in order to stay healthy, I have good news for you: you don't. Matthew's story is exceptional and fascinating, which is why I chose to make it the feature story of this chapter, but I have many, many more examples of people who used a free spiritual practice in the comfort of their own homes in order to get well. That is the beauty of spiritual connection practices: they do not cost anything except your time.

Remember, a spiritual practice is one that encourages you to feel—in your body and your emotions—a deep sensation of calm and peace. In order to feel this, you first have to find a way to shut off your thinking mind. Many people feel spiritual energy very subtly at first, like a gentle wave of calmness—the way you might feel after watching a sunset. If you want to intensify that post-sunset feeling, you will likely have to commit to doing your spiritual practice daily, so the feeling can build up over time.

Here are some ideas of spiritual practices you can try this week:

- *Deep Breathing.* Take a moment right now to put everything aside, close your eyes, and take ten deep inhalations and exhalations. Place your hands on your lower belly while you do this so you can feel your hands rise and fall with your breath. Silently count to ten exhalations, then open your eyes. See if you feel any calmer. If you do, commit to doing this every day for two weeks.

- *Walking Outside.* Take a ten-minute walk outside today, bringing nothing with you except perhaps calming music. Try not to think during this walk; instead, just observe the world around you. If your thinking mind gets restless, try this silent mantra: on your next inhale, say to yourself *I am grate-*

ful for, and on the exhale fill in the blank. Set a timer for ten minutes. If you feel more peaceful after this walk, commit to taking one every day for two weeks.

- *Guided Imagery.* Go to iTunes or your local library and download or borrow a guided imagery CD. Mental imagery is one "trick" for stopping the thinking mind, because it asks the mind to focus on imagery instead of letting it run wild with thoughts. If you feel more peaceful after listening to the guided imagery, commit to listening to it every day for two weeks.

- *Guided Meditation.* Get a guided meditation CD from iTunes or your local library and listen to its instructions. Some of my favorites include Jon Kabat-Zinn and Eckhart Tolle. If you feel more peaceful after listening to the guided meditation, commit to listening to it every day for two weeks.

- *Daily Prayer.* If praying is something that appeals to you, set aside a time each day to pray quietly for at least five minutes. Take deep breaths while you do this, and really try to imagine connecting to a peaceful, divine energy.

- *Spiritual Groups.* Look around your neighborhood for a local spiritual group (e.g., weekly meditation or prayer circle) that has a strong *practice* component to it (as opposed to just listening to a lecture or sermon). Many people find that practicing in a group setting, especially if they are just beginning a spiritual practice, holds them accountable and gives them the support they need to make it a daily habit.

- *Online Groups.* If there are no in-person groups in your neighborhood, you can try joining an online group. Again, look for one that is practice-oriented, where group members are encouraged to check in about how their daily spiritual practice is going.

Remember, a spiritual practice such as these examples listed is not just something you do for your emotional well-being but also for your physical health. When the thinking mind stops and spiritual energy begins to flow through you, a whole host of healthy changes occur in your physical body, including a rush of healthy hormones streaming from your pineal and pituitary glands into your bloodstream, increased oxygenation of the body, improved blood circulation, decreased blood pressure, improved digestion and detoxification, a stronger immune system, and the ability to turn off unhealthy genes. These practices can transform your body for the better in a very powerful way, especially if you practice them daily.

———

RESEARCHERS HAVE COME a long way in discovering the physical effects of a spiritual practice, and I believe that someday they will be able to explain exactly why and how Matthew healed using the spiritual connecting practice of meditation. In the meantime, perhaps the most important concept to take away from this chapter is that spirituality can be a physical, felt experience of unconditional love that results from a daily "connecting" practice, such as meditation, prayer, or even dancing, singing, gardening, etc. In other words, the concept of spirituality does not have to be limited to a set of religious beliefs that one holds in the mind but rather an experience of blissful energy you *feel in your body* as a result of a daily practice. This is why I suggest to cancer patients that they find a connecting practice that works for them—not only because it has been shown to boost the immune system, but simply because it feels really good.

CHAPTER 9

HAVING STRONG
REASONS FOR LIVING

*I don't believe people are looking for the meaning of life as much
as they are looking for the experience of being alive.*

—JOSEPH CAMPBELL

When I was first analyzing the transcripts from the Radical Remission survivors and alternative healers I interviewed during my research trip around the world, I began to notice a recurring factor I initially called "having an 'I don't want to die' attitude." However, as my research continued, I realized that this was not quite the right name for it. While it was true the Radical Remission survivors did not want to die, that was only because they really wanted to keep living—and this is a subtle, yet important, difference.

For example, in my consulting work over the past ten years, I have met many cancer patients who are very afraid of death. These people certainly have a strong "I don't want to die" attitude. However, what I saw in the transcripts was something different: these people did not so much have a fear of death as a zest for living. In fact, a few of them were completely unafraid of death, seeing it as nothing more than a transition to a different existence, which would happen "whenever it was meant to happen." Until it happened, though, these people were very excited about all the things they still wanted to do while they were alive in their bodies. As a result of this subtle difference, I eventually changed the name of this ninth factor.

After taking a look at three important aspects of "having strong reasons for living," we will read the healing story of one woman whose zest for life kept her motivated during her journey with advanced colon cancer. At the end of this chapter, you will find a simple list of action steps that can help put that essential spring back into your step.

CONFIDENCE FROM YOUR CORE

Radical Remission survivors and alternative healers emphasize that a person's desire to live has to come from the deepest core of his or her being, and it has to be unquestioning. The unwavering conviction is "Yes! I want to *keep living.*" There is no doubt in the person's mind that he or she is absolutely excited about life and wants to stay on this earth for as long as possible. One of the alternative healers I studied, a kahuna healer from Hawaii named Serge Kahili King, describes this concept as it relates to fear:

> *It is an experiential fact that you cannot feel fear if your body is totally relaxed. However, even though there are hundreds, if not thousands, of ways to relax—such as massage, meditation, play, laughter, herbs—that does not always solve the problem. The real problem lies* behind *the tension, behind the fear. The real problem is not even the idea that something is fearful. The real problem is that you feel helpless. When this problem [of helplessness] is solved, the fear disappears . . . and a huge amount of*

tension disappears. . . . Fundamentally, what I'm really talk-
ing about is confidence, a kind of core confidence. . . . There is
no quick-and-easy fix I know of that will produce this kind of
confidence. It takes internal awareness and one or more internal
decisions.

Similarly, a longtime cancer survivor who discovered her core
conviction to keep living is Leigh Fortson. Leigh was diagnosed
with anal cancer at the age of forty-eight, when her children were
only ten and twelve. Over the next three years, her cancer unfortunately came back twice, forcing her to seek out complementary
approaches she could integrate into her conventional surgery, radiation, and chemo. Throughout this roller coaster of a journey, her
core conviction of wanting to keep living kept her grounded:

When I first got diagnosed, I was hit with questions about free
will and how much my will had to do with my recovery. At
first, as is typical I think, I thought of my children. They were
the reason I wanted to live. By my second diagnosis, however, it
needed to be about wanting to live for me, *because I wasn't done*
yet. It worked. These days, as I continue to have recoveries and
relapses, I have come to understand that my deepest desire to go
on living is because we were born on purpose: to live life with as
much love as possible. We came to live life to its fullest. Even when
I'm mad at life, every time something difficult happens to me or
someone I love, every time I get pissed off that the tumor and ra-
diation have left me unable to walk far or gracefully, every time I
feel pain because of all that, I ask myself, "Even with this, do you
want to live?" And every time my body feels a subtle jubilation. I
hear "Yes!" from deep within.

It is going on seven years since Leigh's initial diagnosis, and her unwavering will to live gives her the strength she needs to keep searching for new ways to improve her health.

THE MIND LEADS THE BODY

We have seen this second aspect many times throughout this book, but it is worth reiterating: the mind leads the body, not the other way around.

From a scientific standpoint, it is a proven fact that when you have a strong thought or emotion, powerful hormones are released instantly into your bloodstream; they have either a beneficial or detrimental effect on your immune system, depending on the nature of that thought or emotion. From an alternative medicine standpoint, having strong reasons for living invites chi into the body. Similar to inhaling, alternative healers believe that we invite the breath of life into us when we are excited about living, but when we are not excited about being here, we will eventually not bring in enough chi to keep our bodies alive anymore, as chi is the energy that gives life to the body.

One Radical Remission survivor who believes the mind leads the body, and not the other way around, is Glenn Sabin. Driven by his desire to have children and watch them grow up, Glenn created a comprehensive, integrative oncology approach to achieve a complete remission of his CLL (chronic lymphocytic leukemia)—considered an "incurable" disease—without using any conventional interventions such as chemotherapy or bone marrow transplants. During this process, the power that the mind has over the body became one of his most important discoveries:

I was twenty-eight years old and newly married when I was told that I had an incurable form of leukemia that typically strikes

people in their seventies. The choices offered were either an ex-
perimental bone marrow transplant or "watchful waiting"—
essentially waiting for the disease to make the first move. I loved
life so much that, for literally two decades, I painstakingly looked
for answers on how best to position my body and mind to heal.
I have followed a rigorous, evidence-based, integrative oncology
protocol for years, including exercise, supplements, diet, mind-
body exercises, and more—and it has resulted in a complete
remission. Throughout all of this, I have come to believe that
the brain is the most powerful and least understood organ in the
human body. I believe it runs the entire human machine and that
its innate healing capacity is enormous. The healing of any disease
starts with a calm, unfettered mind and a strong desire to live.

Glenn's original diagnosis was more than twenty-two years ago,
and today he considers himself not a cancer survivor but a cancer
"thriver." He and his wife have two children, who are a continual
source of joy and inspiration. His case has been documented by the
Dana-Farber Cancer Institute in Boston and by his oncologist, Lee
M. Nadler, M.D., a dean at Harvard Medical School.

Similar to Glenn, one of the alternative healers I interviewed
from Zimbabwe also believes the mind is a primary shaper in the
health of the physical body. While this healer uses many esoteric
techniques in his shamanic healing work, such as listening to what
his spirit guides tell him about a patient's health status, he feels
strongly that his patients' beliefs are paramount when it comes to
their healing:

I've seen that my [conventional medicine] colleagues sometimes fail
to cure their patients. . . . With that kind of patient, the doctors are
telling [the patients] that they're going to die. But my spirits are tell-

ing me that they're not going to die; they're going to live! . . . What make someone get better is the belief that they're going to live, to get over this problem. When you believe in something in your brain, your whole body accepts that, and then you pour through [i.e., quickly overcome] your problem. But when your brain does not accept you are going to overcome this, then you're definitely dying. It's the strength of the belief of somebody that makes them get better.

According to this African healer, the body listens to what the mind tells it: if the mind is excited about living, the body will be filled with life-giving energy, but if the mind is fearful or hopeless, then the body will be cut off from receiving that essential energy.

FINDING YOUR CALLING

In order to be excited about living, people often need to get in touch with (or get back in touch with) their deepest desires or callings. For many people, this third aspect of "having strong reasons for living" means adding creativity back into their lives, because creativity is something that unfortunately most adults have lost touch with. For example, many people's jobs do not provide them with much of a creative outlet, and their evenings are then filled with cooking, cleaning, perhaps taking care of children, and resting.

A cancer diagnosis, however, is a wake-up call, and that means some people waking up to the fact that they may not be very excited about one or more aspects of their lives, whether it be their careers, romantic relationships, family lives, spiritual lives, communities, or hobbies. Being diagnosed with cancer tends to force people to reflect on what they would ideally like to change in order to make their remaining time on this planet—however long that may be—as enjoyable and meaningful as possible.

One of the longtime survivors I met whose cancer diagnosis allowed her to find her deeper calling is Tami Boehmer. Tami was diagnosed at age thirty-eight with early-stage breast cancer, and when it returned six years later as stage 4 breast cancer, she decided to tackle it with an integrative approach, combining conventional medicine with supplements, exercise, visualization, faith, and a whole-foods diet. However, despite all this, she realized that something was still missing from her life:

> *Despite all I was doing, I began to feel depressed and fearful about dying. Every morning I woke up with the thought,* I have cancer. *I certainly had strong reasons to live: my husband and especially my daughter, who was only nine at the time. I knew I had to be around to raise her. But I needed hope that this was possible, and I was getting just the opposite from doctors. Then I had a kind of epiphany. I decided to write a book about advanced-stage cancer patients and how they beat the odds. I thought it would not only be therapeutic for me but it could help others. The empty hole I was feeling started to dissipate. This was the sense of purpose I was seeking, and it gave me hope that I, too, could beat the odds and be able to nurture my daughter through adulthood.*

Tami's book, *From Incurable to Incredible: Cancer Survivors Who Beat the Odds,* is currently fulfilling her deeper calling to spread hope to others (and herself), while she also focuses on spending quality time with her husband and daughter.

Similar to Tami, Josie RavenWing also emphasizes the importance of developing new life goals in order to keep the body healthy. Josie is an American-born energy healer who now spends most of her time in Brazil. She explains the relationship between life force and having strong reasons for living:

You've heard of the Retirement Syndrome or the Empty Nest Syndrome, where people have planned things out in their life only up to a certain point—like retirement or when their children are grown—and they have no more goals after that. What happens a lot of times if they don't develop [their goals] is that their energy just collapses in on [itself], and often they get ill or they die really soon afterward, at a time when they're supposed to be light and free and enjoying themselves. But they haven't set any goals, and so the life force doesn't have a direction to keep being pulled forward toward something. So, that's why I say the people who still have strong dreams, strong goals of things that they want to do, and who have a strong desire to be well—those can be powerful factors in a faster healing process.

For Josie and many of the other alternative healers I study, having enough goals or projects in your life that excite you is absolutely essential for bringing in enough chi to keep your body healthy and alive.

RESEARCH ON HAVING STRONG REASONS FOR LIVING

Having strong reasons for living means focusing on why you want to keep living instead of the fact that you might die sooner than you had hoped. In some cases, doing this can seem to other people as if you are denying the possibility of death altogether. We often think of "denial" as a negative word; however, when it comes to cancer, studies have shown that a little bit of denial can actually be very healthy for you. For example, a landmark study that followed breast cancer patients for five years showed that women who had an initial reaction of denial toward their cancer were significantly less likely to have recurrences than those who initially reacted with either stoic acceptance or helplessness.[1] Three similar studies have found that high levels of denial are significantly associated with longer survival times in cancer patients.[2] And in a recent study of lung cancer patients, those who had a high level of denial experienced fewer physical side effects compared to those who had low levels of denial.[3] Taken altogether, these studies show us that not focusing on dying, and instead focusing on other things—such as your reasons for living—may actually help you survive cancer longer, reduce your chances of a recurrence, and give you fewer side effects.

While denying death may help you live longer, other studies have shown that being depressed may cause you to die sooner. Depression is characterized by an inability to find joy in one's life; it can therefore be thought of as the *opposite* of having strong reasons for living. Study after study—including one meta-analysis that looked at the results of seventy-six different studies conducted on depression and cancer—have shown that depressed and/or hopeless cancer patients die significantly sooner than non-depressed cancer patients.[4] What's more, this ability for depression to predict mortality in cancer patients holds true regardless of your cancer type or cultural background.[5] These depressed cancer patients are described as saying things like "I just want to give up," which indicates they no longer have strong reasons for living. All in all, these studies imply that depression can lead to a quicker death for cancer patients.

So, the research has shown that denial can help cancer patients live longer, and depression can cause them to die sooner, but what about having strong reasons to live? What can *that* do? That question is a little harder to answer, because not many studies have looked specifically at how this might affect a cancer patient's health. Instead, most studies have looked at something called a "fighting spirit," which is quite different. Having a fighting spirit means you are engaged in a fight against your cancer.[6] Having strong reasons to live does not mean you are necessarily fighting anything; instead, it means you are focused on things that bring you joy, meaning, and happiness. Interestingly, similar studies to my own have also found that Radical Remission survivors exhibit unusually strong reasons for living.[7]

When a cancer patient has a strong "fighting spirit," that focus on fighting can lead to a constant, low-level, fight-or-flight response in the body, which can weaken the immune system and release a steady stream of stress hormones into the bloodstream. To our hunter-gatherer brains, it's like constantly feeling as if we need to be fighting a tiger that's chasing us. I believe this is the main reason that having a "fighting spirit" has *not* been shown to help cancer patients live longer in numerous, well-designed studies.[8] Meanwhile, having strong reasons for living involves focusing on things that bring a person meaning and joy, and this actually turns *off* the fight-or-flight response and turns *on* the rest-and-repair response, which in turn tells the body to release a slew of immune-boosting hormones, such as serotonin, relaxin, oxytocin, dopamine, and endorphins.

There have not, unfortunately, been any studies conducted specifically on whether having strong reasons for living can help cancer patients live longer, but there are two studies that may shed some light on this topic. As I mentioned earlier, depression can be thought of as the opposite of having strong reasons to live. One study showed that using psychotherapeutic techniques to *decrease* cancer patients' depression led to significantly longer survival times.[9] In other words, by strengthening the patients' reasons for living (by decreasing their depression), the researchers were able to extend the patients' lives significantly. This result gives us one tentative indication that having strong reasons to live may indeed help cancer patients live longer.

A second indication comes from a related study on elderly people's (but not cancer patients') will to live. In that study, elderly people who had a stronger will to live survived the longest, regardless of age, gender, or *any previous medical conditions*.[10] In other words, in this study, having strong reasons for living overpowered things like having more illnesses or being older than your peers when it came to who lived the longest. So, while specific studies have not yet been conducted on whether having strong reasons to live may help you heal from cancer specifically, these two related studies seem to point to the fact that having strong reasons for living—as opposed to being depressed or hopeless—may indeed help people live longer in general.

RADICAL REMISSION SURVIVOR "Donna" had two very strong reasons for living: her two grandchildren. Having such a strong desire to be there with her grandchildren as they grew up gave Donna the strength she needed to keep exploring various outside-the-box options for her medically incurable colon cancer. As you read Donna's story, I invite you to reflect upon your own reasons for living. What gets *you* out of bed in the morning? What have you always wanted to do in your life? Put a different way, what would you look back on and regret *not* doing if you knew you were going to die in two years? The answers to these questions are the kinds of deep, soul-level desires that allow Radical Remission survivors to persevere through their healing journeys.

᧡ Donna's Story ᧡

It all came as quite a shock because Donna did not have any warning symptoms. In 2005, she was a vibrant fifty-eight-year-old woman who embraced life, having retired nine months earlier from her lifelong career as a teacher and later as a school principal. She was thoroughly enjoying her retirement, which included spending lots of time with her first grandchild, anticipating the upcoming birth of her second grandchild, and hosting a weekly meditation circle at her home. Then one day, out of the blue, she was overcome with stomach cramps so severe she decided to take herself to the emergency room. As a divorced mother of two grown children and a teacher for over thirty years, Donna was accustomed to making an occasional trip to the emergency room, whether for a child's broken bone or someone's bumped head. What she was not expecting was a doctor telling her that a large tumor was completely blocking her colon and she would need emergency surgery the next morning.

She awoke from that emergency surgery only to hear the devastating news that she had stage 3 colon cancer, confirmed by a biopsy they had done during the surgery. Due to the extensive nature of her cancer, she also awoke with a colostomy bag hanging from her stomach. A colostomy is a surgical procedure in which the colon is diverted into a plastic bag attached to your abdomen, such that you no longer have normal bowel movements. Because her cancer was stage 3, meaning it had spread beyond her colon into many of the surrounding lymph nodes, Donna's doctors told her that, once she recovered from the surgery, she would need immediate chemotherapy. Despite this ominous situation, Donna's naturally optimistic nature kept her from becoming overly scared:

I never got to the point of feeling that things were dire. Not even when I was in the hospital. One of the doctors came and said, "I don't understand it. How come you're not reacting?" . . . I don't know; I just didn't go there. . . . I felt that I still had things to do here—lots of people to meet, places to go. And then there were my children and my grandchildren. . . . It was just never in my mind that I was going to have any problems. . . . I don't know if that's total avoidance or what, but it worked.

Donna's core conviction that she wanted to keep living for as long as possible allowed her to focus fully on recovering from the surgery, and a few weeks later she was ready to begin chemo. However, after only five daily chemotherapy infusions, she found herself in the hospital's intensive care unit (ICU), because her body had stopped making white blood cells. She spent the next six days in the ICU, interspersed with visits from her supportive family and friends, many of whom gave her Reiki healing while she was bedridden.

Her body slowly started making white blood cells again, but her doctors told her that she would not be able to continue with the standard dose of chemotherapy, because her body was clearly unable to tolerate it. They also told her that if they reduced the dose, the chemotherapy would not work. Their only other alternative was an experimental medication, but it had not been very successful in other patients and it was also potentially fatal. So, their final and most viable option was for her simply to go home and get her affairs in order. Luckily, Donna's friend from her weekly meditation circle had a different idea:

After doing five days of [chemo], I looked like I was 105 years old—honest to God! And my hair all fell out and my face was

gray and sunken. I looked like death warmed over. That's
when my friend said, "You have *to go detox this chemo. Go to*
Elisabeth. She'll get this out of your system."

To Donna, who certainly had no intention of getting her affairs
in order but instead wanted to do whatever it took to stay around
for her grandchildren, detoxing sounded like a great alternative. Her
friend explained that Elisabeth Pazdzierski was a local acupuncturist and herbalist who offered ten-day health retreats at a beautiful
nearby lodge called Cougar Mountain Therapy Center. Intrigued,
Donna told her doctors that she wished to decline the potentially
fatal experimental treatment, and she signed up for the next Cougar
Mountain retreat. Another priority for her was finding a way to rein
in her underlying fear of death:

> *For a short, brief time I went,* Oh my God, what if [I die]? *This*
> *was after I was home [from the hospital]. And I was thinking,*
> I've got two sons, and they've got family, and there are the
> grandchildren. *And I'm thinking what if. And then I gave myself*
> *a slap in the face and went,* You're not going anywhere, so
> that's enough of that. Don't even go there. *And I remember my*
> *youngest son saying, "Mom, you're not dealing with your feelings."*
> *And I said to him, "I've already gone there. I've gone to the what*
> *if." And then I was like,* No. I need to take charge of this. I
> need to do what I have to do here. I'm not going *anywhere.*

In other words, Donna purposefully chose to focus on what she
could do to be around for her children and grandchildren, as opposed to the fact that she might die. So, it was with this newfound
determination that she dragged her bald-headed, weak body to the
Cougar Mountain Therapy Center, located in the foothills of the

British Columbia mountains. Her goal was to get the chemotherapy out of her body and then work on building up her immune system. The price was similar to an expensive vacation—about five thousand dollars for ten days, which included all lodging, meals, and treatments. Given that her Western doctors had told her that her days were numbered, she figured it would not hurt to spend some of her savings in this final, Hail Mary attempt at turning her health around. At the very least, she figured she would get a decent vacation out of it:

> *When I went [to Cougar Mountain] I was very, very weak. I couldn't walk very far. I mean I could hardly walk from the house to the gate. By the time I left there, I was walking a couple of kilometers—and I was only there ten days! Elisabeth started out training as a doctor and then decided she would use the holistic approach. And so she uses Chinese medicine, acupuncture, diet. . . . Depending on what needed to be worked on, I would get acupuncture at least once a day, possibly twice.*

In addition to her daily acupuncture treatments, Donna ate the healthy food that was served to her and the other seven guests on the retreat. It was primarily colorful vegan fare along with a bit of fish. This was a big change for Donna, who had been a moderate meat eater and self-proclaimed sugar addict her whole life.

Two other treatments that she tried at Cougar Mountain were a Rife machine and a magnetic pulser. Both of these are popular alternative treatments for cancer patients, although most conventional doctors believe they have no significant effect on cancer cells. Nonetheless, there are numerous anecdotes of cancer patients who have healed after using such machines. They work by emitting small electric impulses at varying frequencies, the theory being that because all atoms vibrate, certain frequencies should cause certain cells (e.g., cancer cells) to "shatter" and die, much like an opera singer can shatter certain glasses by singing a particular note.

Donna also took part in group activities that helped to cultivate a sense of social support among the retreat participants. Plus, the idea of releasing suppressed emotions from the past was explored in one-on-one consultations with Elisabeth:

> Toward the end [of the ten days], Elisabeth and her assistant would do a private session and sort of go, "What is it that either makes you sad or . . . has made you unhappy? Go back into your childhood, and go and see just exactly what it is that's bothering you or what upset you way back when." . . . And [afterward] you kind of went, "Oh, look at that! That's been part of my problem here." And so you identified it.

At the end of the retreat, Donna already felt immensely better. Her sons were amazed that she was now able to walk a full mile and a healthy color had returned to her cheeks and skin. She was thrilled to be able to walk up and hug them with strength and vitality again. Elisabeth sent her home with a detailed grocery list, and with Donna's strong will to live motivating her, she enrolled in a vegetarian cooking class.

After coming home from Cougar Mountain, Donna received a lot of love and support from her two sons, two daughters-in-law, and her one cuddly grandbaby, which buoyed her spirits tremendously. Now that she was feeling stronger, she made it a goal to try to see her children and grandchild at least once a week:

> I just have a very loving family and I wasn't ready to leave anybody. There was no way that I wanted to miss out on the

grandchildren growing up, going to high school, being able to take them to the park or to plays. You know? Grandma's a big part of their life, and they're a big part of my life, so that's that. I've been a teacher, so children are my love. I've always enjoyed being with and taking care of children, so this was just a natural thing for me to want to do. I just had it in my mind that I wanted to take them places.

So, Donna did everything in her power to make sure she would be around to see them grow up, including continuing to receive weekly acupuncture and going on daily, outdoor walks. She also went to see a naturopath, who encouraged her to stay on the no meat, no wheat, no sweets, no dairy Cougar Mountain diet and to start taking two immune-boosting vitamin supplements.

Because Donna had believed for many years before her cancer diagnosis that the mind has a powerful effect on the health of the body, she also made sure to keep her mind focused on her reasons for living, as opposed to on any fearful thoughts that tried to creep in. To accomplish this, she continued with her regular meditation practice and began listening to visualization CDs every night before going to bed. In her opinion, the body follows what the mind is thinking, so thinking about staying healthy for her grandchildren was her top priority:

If you're feeling like you're on your way out, your body will pay attention to what you're telling it. . . . But you can lie to yourself. You can tell yourself anything you want, and your body will react to what you're telling it! So, you tell it that it's healthy. You visualize going through an electrified screen door and destroying cancer cells. You do that on a daily basis, and the body doesn't know any different; it follows what the mind tells it to do. . . .

For me, it was just my refusal to go. You know? I was going, "No, I am not done!"

Taken altogether, Donna was doing a wide variety of things to try to make sure she would be able to see her grandchildren grow up, from staying mentally focused on her strong reasons for living to the exercise, diet change, visualization, supplements, and more. From my point of view as a researcher, I was certainly struck by the absolute certainty in her mind that she was not going to die simply because she had too many things she still wanted to do in her life. This strong desire clearly motivated her to adhere to her new diet, keep taking her supplements, and maintain her daily walking—all of which she continues to this day.

Two years after her doctors sent her home to get her affairs in order, Donna felt so well that she made an appointment with her surgeon to see if she could have her colostomy reversed. To reverse a colostomy, a second surgery is required in which the diverted colon is reconnected to the rest of the colon, so normal bowel functions can resume. Donna's surgeon was quite surprised to see her walk into his office at all, much less be doing so well. After a brief and baffled discussion, he happily agreed to perform the surgery, and she has been living without a colostomy bag ever since.

As she reflects on her life-changing experience of cancer, Donna believes that stress and her love of sugar may have been contributing factors, as well as the fact that she always took care of everyone else before taking care of herself. When she got cancer, however, she made sure to change that habit and start doing all the things that gave *her* meaning and excitement, such as traveling, going out to dinners, and sharing what she has learned about healing with others:

I truly didn't have any problems with the colostomy. I traveled! I
went down to Arizona with my friends, colostomy and all. And
I didn't shy away from going out for dinner. It was like, Okay,
take care of this colostomy. . . . *And I remember thinking,*
This has been a very interesting learning experience. If I
could share this with people, I will do that. . . . *To me, I went*
through this because I can help others. So, it seemed more of a
learning experience than anything else. . . . When I'm asked
to speak to a cancer patient, I tell them that [cancer] is not the
boogie man it's made out to be. There are things that you can do.

It has now been more than eight years since Donna was sent home
from the ICU and told to put her affairs in order. Her zest for life
continues to be infectious, and when I speak with her, it's hard to
believe that I am talking to someone in her sixties, since she sounds
like a thirty-year-old. In my most recent conversation with her, I
asked her how she was doing and how she was spending her time.
She replied with a long list of things that bring her joy and meaning:

I am keeping busy babysitting my now four *grandchildren, hosting*
meditation at my house on Friday evenings, volunteering at the
Red Cross and the Salvation Army, and just enjoying life. I am in
very good health, have good energy, and great family and friends.
Life is an adventure, and I am enjoying every moment! . . . And
I still feel that there are many things for me to do yet, so I'm not
prepared to go yet. I've put the age eighty-eight out there. I think
that at eighty-eight I might be ready to go. I'm sixty-seven now, so
I've got about twenty years to go.

Donna's story is a great example of how even the most life-
threatening situations can be turned around—to go from advanced

colon cancer to a complete remission with a reversed colostomy bag in less than two years is quite extraordinary. Throughout it all, her strong and constant desire to keep living provided her with the life-force energy she needed to try a variety of different healing modalities, which, taken together, led to a complete remission.

Action Steps

If you are like many people these days, boredom and/or depression may be occasional, or constant, companions in your life. Or you may simply have a desire to bring more creativity and vitality into your life after reading this chapter. Regardless of where you stand on the "having strong reasons for living" scale, here are some simple ways you can make your life feel more vibrant and meaningful:

- Write down how many years you want to live. Research conducted on people who live to be one hundred has shown that most of them always knew with deep conviction that they wanted to live to be one hundred. Keep your ideal number taped to your bathroom mirror so you see it every morning as you start your day. Of course, if you ever feel like changing your number, feel free.

- Write your ideal obituary. It may sound morbid, but find a quiet evening to sit down, perhaps light a candle and put on some calming music, and write your ideal obituary (unless, of course, this goes against any religious beliefs you may have). Regardless of your current health status, let this truly be your *ideal* obituary, including the ideal age to which you'd like to live and the ideal way in which you'd like to die or leave your body. Also, write down who ideally would survive you (e.g., children, grandchildren) and what ideally you would like to be remembered for having accomplished. Although this can be a very emotional experience for people (keep tissues handy!), I have found that it is a powerful way to both face one's fear of death and elicit one's deepest desires.

• Make a simple list of all your current reasons for living and enjoying life. Try to do this when you are in a good mood, so you can create a nice long list of all the things that currently bring you meaning and joy. Then put a star next to anything you'd like to increase or have more of in your life. Next, below that list, make another list of anything new you'd like to add to your life in order to bring it more creativity, happiness, and meaning. Then make it a goal to start bringing these things into your life on a more frequent basis.

• Try this powerful, three-step exercise for finding your calling, adapted from an exercise found on the audio CD by Rick Jarow entitled *The Ultimate Anti-Career Guide: The Inner Path to Finding Your Work in the World.* I have found it to be one of the quickest and most powerful ways to get in touch with your deepest calling(s).

   1. Imagine that you have unlimited wealth (say, over three hundred billion dollars), perfect health, and are guaranteed total and complete success in whatever you set out to do. Really let your imagination run wild. Then take out some paper and write down all the things you would do with your life (remember, you are guaranteed wild success!). Be sure to cover things like romantic relationships, family, career, hobbies, housing, travel, community, etc.

   2. On a different day, take out another sheet of paper and imagine that, regardless of your current health status, doctors discover that you are going to die in a year and

a half of a painless stroke that cannot be prevented. Keeping in mind that nothing else about your current life would change (i.e., you don't win the lottery in this scenario), how would you choose to spend your last year and a half? (This part of the exercise can get very emotional, so keep tissues handy.)

3. Send an e-mail to answer@RadicalRemission.com for an explanation of how your responses to these two very different scenarios relate to your deeper calling(s). This exercise works best if you complete parts 1 and 2 before reading the explanation.

––––––––––

ALTHOUGH THIS CHAPTER has focused on having strong reasons for living, I want to state clearly that I don't believe anyone should ever feel guilty about being afraid of death. Sadness and fear are natural human emotions, and almost everyone will experience them deeply at some point in their lives, especially when it comes to facing death. However, as we learned in chapter 5, allowing emotions to flow in, through, and out of us—as opposed to letting them get stuck in our minds and bodies—is vital to our health. What I see in the Radical Remission survivors I study is not necessarily a complete fearlessness about death (although some do have that), but rather enough desire for life that their fear of death does not become all-encompassing. The common thread is a desire to live life for as long as possible, not to avoid death at all costs—and that is an important distinction.

Many Radical Remission survivors have taken some time to look death in the face and accept its inevitability. However, they also re-alize that no one—not even their doctors—can know for sure when they are going to die. So, they decide not to focus on the unpredictable timing of when they will actually leave their bodies; instead, they concentrate on all the things they want to do *while still in* their bodies. In this way, focusing on their reasons for living becomes a welcome distraction from any fear of death they may have.

That is why one of the first questions I always ask cancer patients is "Why do you want to stay alive?" Not just *do* you want to stay alive, but *why*. What else would you still like to experience in this life? Which activities bring you energy and joy? I encourage them—and I encourage you—to consider these questions, because even if we never achieve all our life goals, simply having them allows us to keep pulling invigorating life-force energy into our bodies.

CONCLUSION

He who has health, has hope.
And he who has hope, has everything.
—THOMAS CARLYLE, PHILOSOPHER

As you reflect on this book, I hope you are now convinced that anomalies—that is, rare and unexpected events like Radical Remissions—are worth studying. Throughout history, studying anomalies has led to many important discoveries, including the discovery of penicillin, the x-ray, and the pacemaker. When it comes to the anomaly of Radical Remission, studying such extraordinary healing cases gives us insights into the body's self-healing capability. Simply knowing that a person with stage 4 cancer can become cancer-free without using chemotherapy, radiation, or surgery always leaves me in awe of the body's incredible healing potential.

MULTIFACETED REMISSION

While each chapter in this book contains one healing story that focuses on only one of the nine key factors from my Radical Remission research, this is actually somewhat of a false construct, since all the subjects in this book used sometimes eight, all nine, or even more factors in their healing process. It was never *just one factor* that helped these people get well. This can be quite a frustrating notion for Western medicine researchers, who are accustomed to looking for the one thing that will cure a disease. That would be wonderful, of course, but perhaps the reason why the survivors I research do eight, nine, or more things to overcome their cancer is because both cancer and the body-mind-spirit system are so multifaceted.

We already know that cancer can be caused by toxins, viruses, bacteria, genetic mutation, or cellular breakdown. What makes this already complex disease even more multifaceted is the fact that the state of an individual's body-mind-spirit system plays a pivotal role in whether or not toxins get removed from the body speedily, viruses and bacteria are allowed to take root, genes mutate, or cells break down. The state of the body-mind-spirit system is strongly affected by physical behaviors (e.g., what we eat and drink, how much we exercise and sleep), mental and emotional behaviors (e.g., whether we're experiencing stress or happiness, fear or love), and spiritual behaviors (e.g., whether we feel connected to a deeper source of love, stop our thoughts and relax on a deep level on a regular basis). Given all this complexity, it's no wonder nine—not just one—potential healing factors emerged in my research.

And then there is the wonderful, complex reality of individuality. Radical Remission survivors constantly remind me that no two people on this planet are the same, and therefore no two prescriptions for health will be the same. Some people need to focus more on their diets in order to heal, while others need to focus more on releasing anger from their past. Some need to focus more on taking control of their healing, while others need to focus on detoxifying their bodies with herbal supplements. And some people need to focus on all these things equally. That is why none of the nine key healing factors in this book is more important than the others, because everything depends on which particular factors *your* unique body needs for healing.

EMPOWERMENT

While cancer, the body-mind-spirit system, and the nine key factors of my Radical Remission research may be multifaceted, my goal in writing this book was singular: empowerment. Cancer is currently a devastating disease. Most people feel like they have no power to prevent it, since it so often sneaks up on them without any warning. If diagnosed with cancer, they feel like they also have no power to affect its course, besides whatever their doctors offer them in terms of surgery, chemotherapy, or radiation. If they do manage to go into remission, they then feel powerless in being able to prevent cancer from recurring. Add to that the paralyzing fear of death that comes along with any cancer diagnosis, and we have a nation of 12.5 million disempowered cancer patients,[1] not to mention millions more family and friends who feel powerless to help their loved ones.

That's why I began studying Radical Remissions in the first place. I wanted to take some power back from this very scary disease. After years of in-depth research into this topic, which have culminated in my sharing these nine key factors with you via this book, I now believe there are ways to feel much more powerful when facing cancer—and I hope you do, too. The great thing about these factors is that none of them is rare, hard to access, or prohibitively expensive; instead, all they require is some effort on your part. In addition, they have all been shown to promote health in scientific studies. Finally, they are things you can focus on regardless of whether you

- are trying to prevent cancer,
- have cancer currently and are using Western medicine,

- have cancer currently and have chosen not to use Western medicine, or

- are trying to prevent a cancer recurrence.

Most of the cancer patients I work with say the scariest moment of their journey was the diagnosis, but the second scariest moment was when they went into remission. That's because most cancer survivors are told while in remission that all there is to do is watch and wait to see if the cancer comes back, which is a terrifying and disempowering thing to hear. Now, instead of just watching and waiting, people who are hoping to remain cancer-free can access the power of the nine key factors in this book.

In addition to these factors, there are many more things you can do to improve your health. One of them worth mentioning briefly is exercise. While exercise is certainly among the more than seventy-five healing factors that have emerged in my research, I believe the only reason it didn't become a tenth key factor is because many people are simply too weak to exercise when they first begin their healing journeys. However, as the months go by and they start to heal and feel better, many of them do start to move their bodies, and almost all of them eventually exercise regularly. So, please do not finish this book thinking that moving your body is not important, because it is actually *essential* for your health. Rather, the message from my Radical Remission research is, if you are too sick to exercise at the moment, there is still a path toward healing for you, and on this path you should be able to move your body more each day.

INSPIRATION

What makes Radical Remission cases so inspirational is that they are true: some people with advanced cancer really have found ways to become cancer-free. What's more, Radical Remissions have been documented for almost every type of cancer. These are not anecdotes; they are facts.

For centuries, mountain climbers dreamed of achieving the impossible—climbing the world's tallest mountain—but it wasn't until 1953 that Edmund Hillary and Tenzing Norgay succeeded in summiting Mount Everest. Once that became a fact, they were an inspiration to climbers everywhere, and since then more than 3,500 people have climbed that elusive peak.[2] To me, cases of Radical Remission are similar: I realize that not everyone will be able to climb Mount Everest, just as not every cancer patient will be able to have a Radical Remission, but simply knowing there are people who have achieved that elusive goal of surviving advanced cancer is an extraordinary source of inspiration.

Another thing that inspires me about Radical Remission survivors is how transformational their experiences are for them. Almost all of them say that going through their Radical Remission journey is something they would never take back, since it has led them to transform their lives in such wonderful, health-giving, and loving ways. Of course, most of them wish they hadn't had to go through such suffering in order to achieve that transformation, but nonetheless, the end result is something they now cherish deeply.

Their appreciation of their transformations reminds me of the important difference between curing and healing. Curing means getting rid of a disease, while healing means becoming whole. Curing is sometimes possible, while healing is *always* possible. What I most love about the nine key factors is that they can definitely lead to healing, and for some people, they may also lead to curing. Healing simply means bringing more purpose, happiness, and healthy behaviors into your life, which, in my opinion, are beautiful things to begin right now, regardless of how much time we each have left to live.

NEXT STEPS

In addition to trying some, or all, of this book's nine key healing factors in order to help maintain or regain your health, there are a few next steps I encourage you to take with regard to Radical Remission research.

First, we urgently need to keep collecting and documenting cases of Radical Remission, so we can continue to try to understand how people overcome cancer against all odds. Ideally, we will make it very easy for people to submit their Radical Remission cases to a central, online database shared by both researchers and the general public.

Second, it would be wonderful if these Radical Remission cases could also serve as a source of community and connection between current cancer patients and Radical Remission survivors. Wouldn't it be amazing if, on the night of your breast cancer diagnosis, you could go to a website and read ten, twenty, perhaps even a hundred true healing stories of people who had your exact diagnosis and found a unique way to overcome it?

I deeply hope both of these things will happen. That's why I created this website:

WWW.RADICALREMISSION.COM

On this website, you can (for free):

- *Submit a case of Radical Remission.* Submit either your own healing story or the story of a friend, family member, or patient of yours (as long as you have that person's permission to do so). You may submit your story using a pseudonym, if you would like, and a team of researchers will attempt to verify all cases that are submitted.

- *Search cases of Radical Remission.* Use the search function of the website to find cases of Radical Remission that apply to you. For example, if you are a breast cancer patient with triple negative breast cancer, you can pull up all the Radical Remission cases that we have in our database that match your diagnosis and begin reading healing stories to your heart's content.

So, if you know someone who has had a Radical Remission, please encourage that person to submit his or her healing story to the website, so we can all begin to learn from his or her incredible healing journey.

———

PERHAPS, ONE DAY, scientists will discover a single cure for cancer—a true magic bullet. While we are all waiting for that day to come, I believe one of the best things we can do is make our body-mind-spirit systems as strong as possible, so we can turn on our bodies' own incredible self-healing capabilities. I hope this book has given you some direction on how to do that. And, if you currently have cancer, I hope that by reading this book I will one day be reading your own Radical Remission story.

WWW.RADICALREMISSION.COM

ACKNOWLEDGMENTS

If you've ever written a book, you know it takes a *long* time, a ton of work, and lots and lots of people to make it a reality. I am first and foremost indebted to all the people I have ever interviewed for my research, including all of the Radical Remission survivors and alternative healers mentioned in this book. You are the what, why, and how of this book, and I am forever grateful that you let me into your world of healing. The world is healthier and happier because of what you have shared—thank you.

Also, a huge thank-you to all the people who made my around-the-world research trip possible, including the American Cancer Society, Karin Fuchs, Michaelle Edwards, Dr. David Jin, Bryan McMahon, Chieko Ohori, Catherine Oshida, Blair Sly, Dr. Tsuyoshi Konta, Dan White, Haruka Tsuchiya, the Mimura family, Carolyn Landis, Nan Rick, Swami Brahmdev, Danny, Aleju, Diana, Juanca, Manuela, Claudia, Manu, Andrea, Colin, and everyone else at Aurovalley Ashram, Bill and Barbara Turner, the Stern family, David and Debby Sonnenberg, Marko and Sue Sonnenberg, Morton and Vivian Teich, Neville Hodgkinson, Honour Schram de Jong, Debbie Mwamlima, Dr. Rodwell Vongo, Pete Lungu, Dr. W. Z. Mwale, Bella and Rachel at Tongabezi, Vusa Sibanda, Ophious Sibanda, Irwin and Henri Tjong, Denise and Carlos Sauer, Catherine Tucker, and everyone who visited us at points along the trip.

Deep gratitude to Ned Leavitt, my agent and personal Jambavan—there's no one else I would want in my corner. Thank you and Jillian for believing in my proposal and urging me to come out of my academic shell. And a big thank-you to Kate Northrup for so kindly introducing me to Ned. Thank you to Nancy Hancock, my wonderful editor, who shaped this book into what it is today—I am forever grateful for your belief in and support of this book. And to Elsa Dixon, Suzanne Quist, Melinda Mullin, Amy VanLangen, and everyone else at HarperOne—thank you for putting all of the pieces together to make this happen.

Before it was a book, it was a dissertation, and that would not have been possible without professors Lorraine Midanik, Andrew Scharlach, and Joan Bloom—thank you for supporting my non-traditional research. And to Greg Merrill—you were and continue to be one of the biggest and best mentors of my life. Thank you for encouraging me to know it was okay to carve out my own path, even though it was lonely. Thank you to all the MSW girls and to the now-angel Yolanda Bain for your support while I was at Berkeley, and to Garrett Smith, Lisa Trost, Natalie Ledesma, Julie Argyle, Winnie, Carol, Claudia, and Barbara Buckley, Naomi Hoffer, Paul, and Mimi for guiding me during my early counseling years.

Thank you to Lisa Laing and Dad for our weekly writing calls to keep me on track, and to Sarah Lahey and Mom for reading early drafts. Blessings to the Success Team girls, Steph Cowling and Jennifer Alhasa, for your weekly support and encouragement during the toughest times of writing. And thank you to all of the people who have supported my research and this book from the very beginning with your advice and support and love, including Kate Northrup and Mike Watts, Colleen Saidman and Rodney Yee, Lissa Rankin, Jane Brody, Sara Reistad-Long, Eliot Schrefer, Elyn Jacobs, Ann Fonfa, Glenn Sabin, Murray Jones, Tami Boehmer, Leigh Fortson, Sarto Shickel, Chris Wark, Jeannine Walston, Jan

Adrian, Nancy McKay, Matthew Gilbert, Dale Figtree, Janet Jacobsen, Jim Linderman, Roberta Sorvino, and Lawrence Kuznetz. And a big, gracious, humble thank-you to all the amazing people who wrote endorsements for this book—your words of support mean the world to me.

My research was inspired by other brave authors and researchers who dared to write about Radical Remission before I did, and I am forever grateful for the path these people laid out for me: Caryle Hirschberg, the late Brendan O'Regan, Marilyn Schiltz, and everyone else at IONS, Andrew Weil, Deepak Chopra, Herbert Benson, Anne Harrington, Bernie Siegel, Dean Ornish, Kris Carr, Anita Moorjani, Wayne Dyer, Louise Hay, Rachel Naomi Remen, Bruce Lipton, and Christiane Northrup.

To my friends, whose support I cherish always: the Fontana girls, the Dance Team girls, the Harvard Blocking Group, the SF and Tennis Tuesdays crew, and my New York friends—special shout-out to Jac, Annabelle, Eric, Kim, Rachel, Maiga, Sara, and countless others who were there to support me through the actual writing process—thank you.

To my family, whose love and support grows with each year. Thank you Mom, Dad, Lisa, Andy, Chris, Carrie, Melissa, Sarah, Patrick, and all the nieces and nephews for the love, love, love. Thank you to the best in-laws a gal could hope for—Vivi, Morty, Aly, Karina, Andre, David, Debby, Marko, Sue, Steve, and Howard, and all of your wonderful children—for your unwavering support. A special burst of love to Vivi, who bravely defied the odds of ovarian cancer while I was writing this book. And to our extended family of aunts, uncles, and cousins—thank you for being our own national network of support and fun.

To the baby boy who is currently in my belly and will be in my arms when this book launches—your timing was perfect, we love you so much already, and thank you for your patience during those long hours of editing.

And to my soul mate, Aaron Teich. This book, and the ten years of working, dreaming, studying, agonizing, trip planning, writing, editing, laughing, and crying that went into it, happened only because of you. *Only* because of you. There are simply no words to describe how much you and our marriage mean to me and to my life. I would be lost without you.

And finally, a huge thank-you to you, my readers. I wrote this book to try to help cancer patients and their loved ones in some small way. I hope I succeeded.

FURTHER READING

Battilega, Nancy Ann. 2008. *A Story of Grace: Holistic Healing After a Diagnosis of Breast Cancer*. CreateSpace.

Block, Keith I. 2009. *Life Over Cancer: The Block Center Program for Integrative Cancer Treatment*. New York: Bantam.

Boehmer, Tami. 2010. *From Incurable to Incredible: Cancer Survivors Who Beat the Odds*. CreateSpace.

Bond, Laura. 2013. *Mum's Not Having Chemo: Cutting-Edge Therapies, Real-Life Stories—A Road-Map to Healing from Cancer*. London: Piatkus Books.

Burch, Wanda Easter. 2003. *She Who Dreams: A Journey Into Healing Through Dreamwork*. Novato, CA: New World Library.

Carr, Kris. 2011. *Crazy Sexy Diet: Eat Your Veggies, Ignite Your Spark, and Live Like You Mean It!* Guilford, CT: skirt!

Chopra, Deepak. 1990. *Quantum Healing: Exploring the Frontiers of Mind/Body Medicine*. New York: Bantam.

Cumming, Heather, and Karen Leffler. 2007. *John of God: The Brazilian Healer Who's Touched the Lives of Millions*. New York: Atria.

Figtree, Dale. 2011. *Beyond Cancer Treatment: Clearing and Healing the Underlying Causes: A Personal Memoir and Guide*. Santa Barbara, CA: Blue Palm Press.

Fortson, Leigh. 2011. *Embrace, Release, Heal: An Empowering Guide to Talking About, Thinking About, and Treating Cancer*. Louisville, CO: Sounds True.

Gerson, Charlotte, and Morton Walker. 2001. *The Gerson Therapy: The Proven Nutritional Program for Cancer and Other Illnesses*. New York: Kensington.

Jacobsen, Janet. 2012. *Oh No, Not Another "Growth" Opportunity! An Inspirational Cancer Journey with Humor, Heart, and Healing*. Growth-Ink.

Katz, Rebecca, and Mat Edelson. 2009. *The Cancer-Fighting Kitchen: Nourishing, Big-Flavor Recipes for Cancer Treatment and Recovery*. Berkeley, CA: Ten Speed Press.

Kushi, Michio, and Alex Jack. 2009. *The Cancer Prevention Diet, Revised and Updated Edition: The Macrobiotic Approach to Preventing and Relieving Cancer*. New York: St. Martin's Griffin.

Lipton, Bruce. 2007. *The Biology of Belief: Unleashing the Power of Consciousness, Matter, and Miracles*. Carlsbad, CA: Hay House.

Moorjani, Anita. 2012. *Dying to Be Me: My Journey from Cancer, to Near Death, to True Healing.* Carlsbad, CA: Hay House.

Plant, Jane. 2001. *Your Life in Your Hands: Understanding, Preventing, and Overcoming Breast Cancer.* New York: Thomas Dunne Books.

Quillin, Patrick. 2005. *Beating Cancer with Nutrition.* Carlsbad, CA: Nutrition Times Press.

Rankin, Lissa. 2013. *Mind Over Medicine: Scientific Proof That You Can Heal Yourself.* Carlsbad, CA: Hay House.

RavenWing, Josie. 2002. *The Book of Miracles: The Healing Work of Joao de Deus.* Bloomington, IN: AuthorHouse.

Remen, Rachel Naomi. 1997. *Kitchen Table Wisdom: Stories That Heal.* New York: Riverhead.

Sabin, Glenn. *N-of-1: How One Man's Triumph Over Terminal Cancer Is Changing the Medical Establishment.*

Servan-Schreiber, David. 2009. *Anti-Cancer: A New Way of Life.* New York: Viking.

Schickel, Sarto. 2012. *Cancer Healing Odyssey: My Wife's Remarkable Journey with Love, Medicine, and Natural Therapies.* Pennsylvania: Paxdieta Books.

Siegel, Bernie S. 1998. *Love, Medicine and Miracles: Lessons Learned About Self-Healing from a Surgeon's Experience with Exceptional Patients.* New York: William Morrow.

Somers, Suzanne. 2010. *Knockout: Interviews with Doctors Who Are Curing Cancer—And How to Prevent Getting It in the First Place.* New York: Harmony.

Wark, Chris. Blog: www.christbeatcancer.com.

Weil, Andrew. 2000. *Spontaneous Healing: How to Discover and Embrace Your Body's Natural Ability to Maintain and Heal Itself.* New York: Ballantine Books.

NOTES

INTRODUCTION

1. American Cancer Society, "Pancreatic Cancer Survival by Stage," http://www.cancer .org/cancer/pancreaticcancer/detailedguide/pancreatic-cancer-survival-rates, accessed September 11, 2013.

CHAPTER 1: RADICALLY CHANGING YOUR DIET

1. K. M. Adams et al., "Nutrition in Medicine: Nutrition Education for Medical Students and Residents," *Nutrition in Clinical Practice: Official Publication of the American Society for Parenteral and Enteral Nutrition* 25, no. 5 (October 2010): 471–80.

2. O. Warburg, *The Metabolism of Tumors* (London: Constable, 1930); O. Warburg, "On the Origin of Cancer Cells," *Science* 123, no. 3191 (February 24, 1956): 309–14.

3. R. K. Johnson et al., "Dietary Sugars Intake and Cardiovascular Health: A Scientific Statement from the American Heart Association," *Circulation* 120, no. 11 (September 15, 2009): 1011–20.

4. G. E. Dunaif and T. C. Campbell, "Relative Contribution of Dietary Protein Level and Aflatoxin B1 Dose in Generation of Presumptive Preneoplastic Foci in Rat Liver," *Journal of the National Cancer Institute* 78, no. 2 (February 1987): 365–69; L. D. Youngman and T. C. Campbell, "Inhibition of Aflatoxin B1-Induced Gamma-Glutamyltranspeptidase Positive (GGT+) Hepatic Preneoplastic Foci and Tumors by Low Protein Diets: Evidence that Altered GGT+ Foci Indicate Neoplastic Potential," *Carcinogenesis* 13, no. 9 (September 1992): 1607–13.

5. L. Q. Qin, K. He, and J. Y. Xu, "Milk Consumption and Circulating Insulin-Like Growth Factor-I Level: A Systematic Literature Review," *International Journal of Food Sciences and Nutrition* 60, supplement 7 (2009): 330–40; I. Bruchim and H. Werner, "Targeting IGF-1 Signaling Pathways in Gynecologic Malignancies," *Expert Opinion on Therapeutic Targets* 17, no. 3 (March 2013): 307–20; H. Werner and I. Bruchim, "IGF-1 and BRCA1 Signalling Pathways in Familial Cancer," *The Lancet Oncology* 13, no. 12 (December 2012): e537–44.

6. F. Leiber et al., "A Study on the Causes for the Elevated N-3 Fatty Acids in Cows' Milk of Alpine Origin," *Lipids* 40, no. 2 (February 2005): 191–202; D. F. Hebeisen et al., "Increased Concentrations of Omega-3 Fatty Acids in Milk and Platelet Rich Plasma of Grass-Fed Cows," *International Journal for Vitamin and Nutrition Research (Internationale Zeitschrift für Vitamin- und Ernährungsforschung; Journal International de Vitaminologie et de Nutrition)* 63, no. 3 (1993): 229–33.

7. M. de Lorgeril and P. Salen, "New Insights into the Health Effects of Dietary Saturated and Omega-6 and Omega-3 Polyunsaturated Fatty Acids," *BMC Medicine* 10 (May 2012): 50; A. P. Simopoulos, "The Importance of the Omega-6/Omega-3 Fatty Acid Ratio in Cardiovascular Disease and Other Chronic Diseases," *Experimental Biology and Medicine* 233, no. 6 (June 2008): 674–88.

8. U.S. Department of Agriculture, *Agriculture Fact Book 2001–2002* (Washington, DC: U.S. Government Printing Office, 2003); G. Block, "Foods Contributing to Energy Intake in the U.S.: Data from NHANES 1999–2000," *Journal of Food Composition and Analysis* 17, no. 3–4 (June–August 2004): 439–47.

9. M. Salehi et al., "Meat, Fish, and Esophageal Cancer Risk: A Systematic Review and Dose-Response Meta-Analysis," *Nutrition Reviews* 71, no. 5 (May 2013): 257–67; L. N. Kolonel, "Nutrition and Prostate Cancer," *Cancer Causes and Control* 7, no. 1 (January 1996): 83–94; G. R. Howe and J. D. Burch, "Nutrition and Pancreatic Cancer," *Cancer Causes and Control* 7, no. 1 (January 1996): 69–82; M. T. Goodman et al., "Diet, Body Size, Physical Activity, and the Risk of Endometrial Cancer," *Cancer Research* 57, no. 22 (November 15, 1997): 5077–85; E. Destefani et al., "Meat Intake, Heterocyclic Amines and Risk of Colorectal Cancer," *International Journal of Oncology* 10, no. 3 (March 1997): 573–80; H. Chen et al., "Dietary Patterns and Adenocarcinoma of the Esophagus and Distal Stomach," *American Journal of Clinical Nutrition* 75, no. 1 (January 2002): 137–44; D. S. Chan et al., "Red and Processed Meat and Colorectal Cancer Incidence: Meta-Analysis of Prospective Studies," *PLOS ONE* 6, no. 6 (2011): e20456; L. M. Brown et al., "Dietary Factors and the Risk of Squamous Cell Esophageal Cancer Among Black and White Men in the United States," *Cancer Causes and Control* 9, no. 5 (October 1998): 467–74; C. Bosetti et al., "Diet and Ovarian Cancer Risk: A Case-Control Study in Italy," *International Journal of Cancer (Journal International du Cancer)* 93, no. 6 (September 2001): 911–15; C. Bosetti et al., "Food Groups and Laryngeal Cancer Risk: A Case-Control Study from Italy and Switzerland," *International Journal of Cancer (Journal International du Cancer)* 100, no. 3 (July 2002): 355–60; M. C. Alavanja et al., "Lung Cancer Risk and Red Meat Consumption Among Iowa Women," *Lung Cancer* 34, no. 1 (October 2001): 37–46; W. S. Yang et al., "Meat Consumption and Risk of Lung Cancer: Evidence from Observational Studies," *Annals of Oncology* 23, no. 12 (December 2012): 3163–70.

10. J. R. Hebert, T. G. Hurley, and Y. Ma, "The Effect of Dietary Exposures on Recurrence and Mortality in Early Stage Breast Cancer," *Breast Cancer Research and Treatment* 51, no. 1 (September 1998): 17–28.

11. M. J. Gunter and M. F. Leitzmann, "Obesity and Colorectal Cancer: Epidemiology, Mechanisms and Candidate Genes," *Journal of Nutritional Biochemistry* 17, no. 3 (March 2006): 145–56; E. Giovannucci, "Metabolic Syndrome, Hyperinsulinemia, and Colon Cancer: A Review," *American Journal of Clinical Nutrition* 86, no. 3 (September 2007): s836–42; A. A. Siddiqui, "Metabolic Syndrome and Its Association with Colorectal Cancer: A Review," *American Journal of the Medical Sciences* 341, no. 3 (March 2011): 227–31.

12. Q. Sun et al., "White Rice, Brown Rice, and Risk of Type 2 Diabetes in U.S. Men and Women," *Archives of Internal Medicine* 170, no. 11 (June 14, 2010): 961–69.

13. A. Schatzkin et al., "Dietary Fiber and Whole-Grain Consumption in Relation to Colorectal Cancer in the NIH-AARP Diet and Health Study," *American Journal of Clinical Nutrition* 85, no. 5 (May 2007): 1353–60; D. R. Jacobs Jr., L. F. Andersen, and R. Blomhoff, "Whole-Grain Consumption Is Associated with a Reduced Risk of Noncardiovascular, Noncancer Death Attributed to Inflammatory Diseases in the Iowa Women's Health Study," *American Journal of Clinical Nutrition* 85, no. 6 (June 2007): 1606–14; L. Strayer et al., "Dietary Carbohydrate, Glycemic Index, and Glycemic Load and the Risk of Colorectal Cancer in the BCDDP Cohort," *Cancer Causes and Control* 18, no. 8 (October 3, 2007): 853–63.

14. G. A. Burdock, "Safety Assessment of Castoreum Extract as a Food Ingredient," *International Journal of Toxicology* 26, no. 1 (January/February 2007): 51–55.

15. U.S. Food and Drug Administration, "Code of Federal Regulations: Animal Foods; Labeling of Spices, Flavorings, Colorings, and Chemical Preservatives," in *Title 21-Food and Drugs, Chapter 1, Subchapter E, Part 501, Subpart B, Section 501.22,* 21CRF501.22 ed. (Washington, DC: U.S. Food and Drug Administration: 2013).

16. Centers for Disease Control and Prevention, *Leading Causes of Death, 1900–1998,* http://www.cdc.gov/nchs/data/dvs/lead1900_98.pdf.

17. G. Block, B. Patterson, and A. Subar, "Fruit, Vegetables, and Cancer Prevention: A Review of the Epidemiological Evidence," *Nutrition and Cancer* 18, no. 1 (1992): 1–29; H. Vainio and E. Weiderpass, "Fruit and Vegetables in Cancer Prevention," *Nutrition and Cancer* 54, no. 1 (2006): 111–42.

18. J. A. Meyerhardt et al., "Association of Dietary Patterns with Cancer Recurrence and Survival in Patients with Stage III Colon Cancer," *Journal of the American Medical Association* 298, no. 7 (August 15, 2007): 754–64; J. Ligibel, "Lifestyle Factors in Cancer Survivorship," *Journal of Clinical Oncology* 30, no. 30 (October 20, 2012): 3697–704; C. L. Rock and W. Demark-Wahnefried, "Can Lifestyle Modification Increase Survival in Women Diagnosed with Breast Cancer?" *Journal of Nutrition* 132, no. 11 supplement (November 2002): 3504S–7S; J. P. Pierce, "Diet and Breast Cancer Prognosis: Making Sense of the Women's Healthy Eating and Living and Women's Intervention Nutrition Study Trials," *Current Opinion in Obstetrics and Gynecology* 21, no. 1 (February 2009): 86–91.

19. J. P. Pierce et al., "Greater Survival After Breast Cancer in Physically Active Women with High Vegetable-Fruit Intake Regardless of Obesity," *Journal of Clinical Oncology* 25, no. 17 (June 2007): 2345–51.

20. S. J. Jackson and K. W. Singletary, "Sulforaphane Inhibits Human MCF-7 Mammary Cancer Cell Mitotic Progression and Tubulin Polymerization," *Journal of Nutrition* 134, no. 9 (September 2004): 2229–36.

21. Q. Meng et al., "Suppression of Breast Cancer Invasion and Migration by Indole-3-Carbinol: Associated with Up-Regulation of BRCA1 and E-Cadherin/Catenin Complexes," *Journal of Molecular Medicine (Berlin)* 78, no. 3 (2000): 155–65.

22. Z. Dong, "Effects of Food Factors on Signal Transduction Pathways," *BioFactors* 12, nos. 1–4 (2000): 17–28.

23. F. Vinson et al., "Exposure to Pesticides and Risk of Childhood Cancer: A Meta-Analysis of Recent Epidemiological Studies," *Occupational and Environmental Medicine* 68, no. 9 (September 2011): 694–702.

24. F. Falck Jr. et al., "Pesticides and Polychlorinated Biphenyl Residues in Human Breast Lipids and Their Relation to Breast Cancer," *Archives of Environmental Health* 47, no. 2 (March/April 1992): 143–46.

25. C. Smith-Spangler et al., "Are Organic Foods Safer or Healthier than Conventional Alternatives? A Systematic Review," *Annals of Internal Medicine* 157, no. 5 (September 4, 2012): 348–66.

26. C. Lee and V. D. Longo, "Fasting vs. Dietary Restriction in Cellular Protection and Cancer Treatment: From Model Organisms to Patients," *Oncogene* 30, no. 30 (July 28, 2011): 3305–16.

27. G. R. van den Brink et al., "Feed a Cold, Starve a Fever?" *Clinical and Diagnostic Laboratory Immunology* 9, no. 1 (January 2002): 182–83.

28. L. Raffaghello et al., "Starvation-Dependent Differential Stress Resistance Protects Normal but Not Cancer Cells Against High-Dose Chemotherapy," *Proceedings of the National Academy of Sciences of the United States of America* 105, no. 24 (June 17, 2008): 8215–20; C. Lee and V. D. Longo, "Fasting vs. Dietary Restriction in Cellular Protection and Cancer Treatment: From Model Organisms to Patients," *Oncogene* 30, no. 30 (July 28, 2011): 3305–16; G. R. van den Brink et al., "Feed a Cold, Starve a Fever?" *Clinical and Diagnostic Laboratory Immunology* 9, no. 1 (January 2002): 182–83.

29. M. R. Ponisovskiy, "Warburg Effect Mechanism as the Target for Theoretical Substantiation of a New Potential Cancer Treatment," *Critical Reviews in Eukaryotic Gene Expression* 21, no. 1 (2011): 13–28.

30. N. Krieger et al., "Breast Cancer and Serum Organochlorines: A Prospective Study Among White, Black, and Asian Women," *Journal of the National Cancer Institute* 86, no. 8 (April 20, 1994): 589–99; E. B. Bassin et al., "Age-Specific Fluoride Exposure in Drinking Water and Osteosarcoma (United States)," *Cancer Causes and Control* 17, no. 4 (May 2006): 421–28; O. I. Alatise and G. N. Schrauzer, "Lead Exposure: A Contributing Cause of the Current Breast Cancer Epidemic in Nigerian Women," *Biological Trace Element Research* 136, no. 2 (August 2010): 127–39.

31. J. Lapointe et al., "Gene Expression Profiling Identifies Clinically Relevant Subtypes of Prostate Cancer," *Proceedings of the National Academy of Sciences of the United States of America* 101, no. 3 (January 20, 2004): 811–16.

32. M. C. Bosland et al., "Effect of Soy Protein Isolate Supplementation on Biochemical Recurrence of Prostate Cancer After Radical Prostatectomy: A Randomized Trial," *Journal of the American Medical Association* 310, no. 2 (July 10, 2013): 170–78.

CHAPTER 2: TAKING CONTROL OF YOUR HEALTH

1. L. Temoshok et al., "The Relationship of Psychosocial Factors to Prognostic Indicators in Cutaneous Malignant Melanoma," *Journal of Psychosomatic Research* 29, no. 2 (1985): 139–53.

2. M. Watson et al., "Influence of Psychological Response on Breast Cancer Survival: Ten-Year Follow-Up of a Population-Based Cohort," *European Journal of Cancer* 41, no. 12 (August 2005): 1710–14.

3. P. C. Roud, "Psychosocial Variables Associated with the Exceptional Survival of Patients with Advanced Malignant Disease," *Journal of the National Medical Association* 79, no. 1 (January 1987): 97–102.

4. R. Huebscher, "Spontaneous Remission of Cancer: An Example of Health Promotion," *Nurse Practitioner Forum* 3, no. 4 (December 1992): 228–35.

5. J. N. Schilder et al., "Psychological Changes Preceding Spontaneous Remission of Cancer," *Clinical Case Studies* 3, no. 4 (October 2004): 288–312.

6. A. J. Cunningham et al., "A Prospective, Longitudinal Study of the Relationship of Psychological Work to Duration of Survival in Patients with Metastatic Cancer," *Psycho-oncology* 9, no. 4 (July/August 2000): 323–39.

7. A. J. Cunningham and K. Watson, "How Psychological Therapy May Prolong Survival in Cancer Patients: New Evidence and a Simple Theory," *Integrative Cancer Therapies* 3, no. 3 (September 2004): 214–29.

8. L. S. Katz and S. Epstein, "The Relation of Cancer-Prone Personality to Exceptional Recovery from Cancer: A Preliminary Study," *Advances in Mind-Body Medicine* 21, nos. 3–4 (Fall/Winter 2005): 6–20.

9. C. Lee and V. D. Longo, "Fasting vs. Dietary Restriction in Cellular Protection and Cancer Treatment: From Model Organisms to Patients," *Oncogene* 30, no. 30 (July 28, 2011): 3305–16.

10. P. Slater and N. Mann, "Why Do the Females of Many Bird Species Sing in the Tropics?" *Journal of Avian Biology* 35, no. 4 (July 2004): 289–94.

11. M. E. Falagas, E. Zarkadoulia, and P. I. Rafailidis, "The Therapeutic Effect of Balneotherapy: Evaluation of the Evidence from Randomised Controlled Trials," *International Journal of Clinical Practice* 63, no. 7 (July 2009): 1068–84; A. Fioravanti et al., "Mechanisms of Action of Spa Therapies in Rheumatic Diseases: What Scientific Evidence Is There?" *Rheumatology International* 31, no. 1 (January 2011): 1–8.

CHAPTER 3: FOLLOWING YOUR INTUITION

1. "More Colour, Less Odour: Smell, Vision and Genes," *The Economist* (U.S.), July 26, 2003.
2. Wanda Easter Burch, *She Who Dreams* (Novato, CA: New World Library, 2003), http://www.newworldlibrary.com.
3. Nancy A. Battilega, *A Story of Grace: Holistic Healing After a Diagnosis of Breast Cancer* (Centennial, CO: Nancy A. Battilega, 2008).
4. R. W. Sperry, "Cerebral Organization and Behavior: The Split Brain Behaves in Many Respects Like Two Separate Brains, Providing New Research Possibilities," *Science* 133, no. 3466 (1961): 1749–57; A. G. Sanfey and L. J. Chang, "Of Two Minds When Making a Decision," *Scientific American* online, June 3, 2008.
5. M. Gershon, *The Second Brain: The Scientific Basis of Gut Instinct and a Ground-breaking New Understanding of Nervous Disorders of the Stomach and Intestines,* 1st ed. (New York: Harper, 1998).
6. A. Bechara et al., "Deciding Advantageously Before Knowing the Advantageous Strategy," *Science* 275, no. 5304 (February 28, 1997): 1293–95.
7. D. J. Bem, "Feeling the Future: Experimental Evidence for Anomalous Retroactive Influences on Cognition and Affect," *Journal of Personality and Social Psychology* 100, no. 3 (March 2011): 407–25.
8. A. Dijksterhuis et al., "On Making the Right Choice: The Deliberation-Without-Attention Effect," *Science* 311, no. 5763 (February 17, 2006): 1005–7.
9. A. Dijksterhuis, "Think Different: The Merits of Unconscious Thought in Preference Development and Decision Making," *Journal of Personality and Social Psychology* 87, no. 5 (November 2004): 586–98.
10. M. Seto et al., "Site-Specific Phonon Density of States Discerned Using Electronic States," *Physical Review Letters* 91, no. 18 (October 31, 2003): 185505.

CHAPTER 4: USING HERBS AND SUPPLEMENTS

1. P. S. Moore and Y. Chang, "Why Do Viruses Cause Cancer? Highlights of the First Century of Human Tumour Virology," *Nature Reviews: Cancer* 10, no. 12 (December 2010): 878–89; K. Alibek, A. Kakpenova, and Y. Baiken, "Role of Infectious Agents in the Carcinogenesis of Brain and Head and Neck Cancers," *Infectious Agents and Cancer* 8, no. 1 (February 2, 2013): 7.
2. C. Castillo-Duran and F. Cassorla, "Trace Minerals in Human Growth and Development," *Journal of Pediatric Endocrinology and Metabolism* 12, no. 5, supplement 2 (September/October 1999): 589–601.
3. D. R. Davis, M. D. Epp, and H. D. Riordan, "Changes in USDA Food Composition Data for Forty-Three Garden Crops, 1950 to 1999," *Journal of the American College of Nutrition* 23, no. 6 (December 2004): 669–82; D. R. Davis, "Declining Fruit and Vegetable Nutrient Composition: What Is the Evidence?" *HortScience* 44, no. 1 (February 2009): 15–19.
4. E. Koh, S. Charoenprasert, and A. E. Mitchell, "Effect of Organic and Conventional Cropping Systems on Ascorbic Acid, Vitamin C, Flavonoids, Nitrate, and

Oxalate in Twenty-Seven Varieties of Spinach (Spinacia Oleracea L.)," *Journal of Agricultural and Food Chemistry* 60, no. 12 (March 28, 2012): 3144–50; J. P. Reganold et al., "Fruit and Soil Quality of Organic and Conventional Strawberry Agroecosystems," *PLOS ONE* 5, no. 9 (2010): e12346.

5. C. Smith-Spangler et al., "Are Organic Foods Safer or Healthier than Conventional Alternatives? A Systematic Review," *Annals of Internal Medicine* 157, no. 5 (September 4, 2012): 348–66.

6. A. Das, N. L. Banik, and S. K. Ray, "Retinoids Induce Differentiation and Down-regulate Telomerase Activity and N-Myc to Increase Sensitivity to Flavonoids for Apoptosis in Human Malignant Neuroblastoma SH-SY5Y Cells," *International Journal of Oncology* 34, no. 3 (March 2009): 757–65; T. C. Hsieh and J. M. Wu, "Targeting CWR22Rv1 Prostate Cancer Cell Proliferation and Gene Expression by Combinations of the Phytochemicals EGCG, Genistein and Quercetin," *Anticancer Research* 29, no. 10 (October 2009): 4025–32; S. Bettuzzi et al., "Chemoprevention of Human Prostate Cancer by Oral Administration of Green Tea Catechins in Volunteers with High-Grade Prostate Intraepithelial Neoplasia: A Preliminary Report from a One-Year Proof-of-Principle Study," *Cancer Research* 66, no. 2 (January 15, 2006): 1234–40; Y. Qiao et al., "Cell Growth Inhibition and Gene Expression Regulation by (-)-Epigallocatechin-3-Gallate in Human Cervical Cancer Cells," *Archives of Pharmacal Research* 32, no. 9 (September 2009): 1309–15; B. J. Philips et al., "Induction of Apoptosis in Human Bladder Cancer Cells by Green Tea Catechins," *Biomedical Research* 30, no. 4 (August 2009): 207–15.

7. C. J. Torkelson et al., "Phase 1 Clinical Trial of Trametes Versicolor in Women with Breast Cancer," *ISRN Oncology* 2012, article 251632 (2012); L. J. Standish et al., "Trametes Versicolor Mushroom Immune Therapy in Breast Cancer," *Journal of the Society for Integrative Oncology* 6, no. 3 (Summer 2008): 122–28.

8. N. Mikirova et al., "Effect of High-Dose Intravenous Vitamin C on Inflammation in Cancer Patients," *Journal of Translational Medicine* 10 (September 11, 2012): 189.

9. S. C. Gupta, S. Patchva, and B. B. Aggarwal, "Therapeutic Roles of Curcumin: Lessons Learned from Clinical Trials," *AAPS Journal* 15, no. 1 (January 2013): 195–218.

10. Z. Liu et al., "Randomised Clinical Trial: The Effects of Perioperative Probiotic Treatment on Barrier Function and Post-Operative Infectious Complications in Colorectal Cancer Surgery, a Double-Blind Study," *Alimentary Pharmacology and Therapeutics* 33, no. 1 (January 2011): 50–63; L. Gianotti et al., "A Randomized Double-Blind Trial on Perioperative Administration of Probiotics in Colorectal Cancer Patients," *World Journal of Gastroenterology* 16, no. 2 (January 14, 2010): 167–75.

11. J. M. Gaziano et al., "Multivitamins in the Prevention of Cancer in Men: The Physicians' Health Study II Randomized Controlled Trial," *Journal of the American Medical Association* 308, no. 18 (November 14, 2012): 1871–80.

12. R. H. Fletcher and K. M. Fairfield, "Vitamins for Chronic Disease Prevention in Adults: Clinical Applications," *Journal of the American Medical Association* 287, no. 23 (June 19, 2002): 3127–29.

CHAPTER 5: RELEASING SUPPRESSED EMOTIONS

1. H. Ohgaki and P. Kleihues, "Population-Based Studies on Incidence, Survival Rates, and Genetic Alterations in Astrocytic and Oligodendroglial Gliomas," *Journal of Neuropathology and Experimental Neurology* 64, no. 6 (June 2005): 479–89.

2. S. Cohen, D. Tyrrell, and A. Smith, "Psychological Stress and Susceptibility to the Common Cold," *New England Journal of Medicine* 325, no. 9 (1991): 606–12.

3. C. B. Pert, *Molecules of Emotion: Why You Feel the Way You Feel* (New York: Scribner, 1997).

4. M. Yu, "Somatic Mitochondrial DNA Mutations in Human Cancers," *Advances in Clinical Chemistry* 57 (2012): 99–138; M. Yu, "Generation, Function and Diagnostic Value of Mitochondrial DNA Copy Number Alterations in Human Cancers," *Life Sciences* 89, nos. 3–4 (July 18, 2011): 65–71; A. Schulze and A. L. Harris, "How Cancer Metabolism Is Tuned for Proliferation and Vulnerable to Disruption," *Nature* 491, no. 7424 (November 15, 2012): 364–73.

5. B. A. McGregor et al., "Cognitive-Behavioral Stress Management Increases Benefit Finding and Immune Function Among Women with Early-Stage Breast Cancer," *Journal of Psychosomatic Research* 56, no. 1 (January 2004): 1–8.

6. F. I. Fawzy et al., "Malignant Melanoma: Effects of an Early Structured Psychiatric Intervention, Coping, and Affective State on Recurrence and Survival Six Years Later," *Archives of General Psychiatry* 50, no. 9 (September 1993): 681–89.

7. J. W. Fielding et al., "An Interim Report of a Prospective, Randomized, Controlled Study of Adjuvant Chemotherapy in Operable Gastric Cancer: British Stomach Cancer Group," *World Journal of Surgery* 7, no. 3 (May 1983): 390–99.

8. S. C. Segerstrom et al., "Worry Affects the Immune Response to Phobic Fear," *Brain, Behavior, and Immunity* 13, no. 2 (June 1999): 80–92.

CHAPTER 6: INCREASING POSITIVE EMOTIONS

1. V. N. Salimpoor et al., "Anatomically Distinct Dopamine Release During Anticipation and Experience of Peak Emotion to Music," *Nature Neuroscience* 14, no. 2 (February 2011): 257–62; J. Burgdorf and J. Panksepp, "The Neurobiology of Positive Emotions," *Neuroscience and Biobehavioral Reviews* 30, no. 2 (2006): 173–87; E. E. Benarroch, "Oxytocin and Vasopressin: Social Neuropeptides with Complex Neuromodulatory Functions," *Neurology* 80, no. 16 (April 16, 2013): 1521–28.

2. L. S. Berk et al., "Modulation of Neuroimmune Parameters During the Eustress of Humor-Associated Mirthful Laughter," *Alternative Therapies in Health and Medicine* 7, no. 2 (March 2001): 62–72, 74–76; M. P. Bennett and C. A. Lengacher, "Humor and Laughter May Influence Health: I. History and Background," *Evidence-Based Complementary and Alternative Medicine: eCAM* 3, no. 1 (March 2006): 61–63; J. Wilkins and A. J. Eisenbraun, "Humor Theories and the Physi-

ological Benefits of Laughter," *Advances in Mind-Body Medicine* 24, no. 2 (Summer 2009): 8–12; L. S. Berk et al., "Neuroendocrine and Stress Hormone Changes During Mirthful Laughter," *American Journal of the Medical Sciences* 298, no. 6 (December 1989): 390–96; S. Cohen et al., "Positive Emotional Style Predicts Resistance to Illness After Experimental Exposure to Rhinovirus or Influenza A Virus," *Psychosomatic Medicine* 68, no. 6 (November/December 2006): 809–15.

3. D. K. Sarkar et al., "Regulation of Cancer Progression by Beta-Endorphin Neuron," *Cancer Research* 72, no. 4 (February 15, 2012): 836–40; E. Ames and W. J. Murphy, "Advantages and Clinical Applications of Natural Killer Cells in Cancer Immunotherapy," *Cancer Immunology, Immunotherapy,* published online August 30, 2013, doi: 10.1007/s00262-013-1469-8; E. Ileana, S. Champiat, and J. C. Soria, "Immune-Checkpoints: The New Anti-Cancer Immunotherapies" (article in French), *Bulletin du Cancer* 100, no. 6 (June 2013): 601–10.

4. Y. Sakai et al., "A Trial of Improvement of Immunity in Cancer Patients by Laughter Therapy," *Japan-Hospitals: The Journal of the Japan Hospital Association* 32 (July 2013): 53–59.

5. S. M. Lamers et al., "The Impact of Emotional Well-Being on Long-Term Recovery and Survival in Physical Illness: A Meta-Analysis," *Journal of Behavioral Medicine* 35, no. 5 (October 2012): 538–47; Y. Chida and A. Steptoe, "Positive Psychological Well-Being and Mortality: A Quantitative Review of Prospective Observational Studies," *Psychosomatic Medicine* 70, no. 7 (September 2008): 741–56.

6. D. K. Sarkar et al., "Regulation of Cancer Progression by Beta-Endorphin Neuron," *Cancer Research* 72, no. 4 (February 15, 2012): 836–40.

7. D. Ornish et al., "Intensive Lifestyle Changes May Affect the Progression of Prostate Cancer," *Journal of Urology* 174, no. 3 (September 2005): 1065–69, discussion 1069–70.

8. D. Ornish et al., "Changes in Prostate Gene Expression in Men Undergoing an Intensive Nutrition and Lifestyle Intervention," *Proceedings of the National Academy of Sciences* 105, no. 24 (June 17, 2008): 8369–74.

9. R. C. Kessler et al., "Prevalence, Severity, and Comorbidity of Twelve-Month DSM-IV Disorders in the National Comorbidity Survey Replication," *Archives of General Psychiatry* 62, no. 6 (June 2005): 617–27.

CHAPTER 7: EMBRACING SOCIAL SUPPORT

1. W. W. Ishak, M. Kahloon, and H. Fakhry, "Oxytocin Role in Enhancing Well-Being: A Literature Review," *Journal of Affective Disorders* 130, nos. 1–2 (April 2011): 1–9.

2. A. Steptoe, S. Dockray, and J. Wardle, "Positive Affect and Psychobiological Processes Relevant to Health," *Journal of Personality* 77, no. 6 (December 2009): 1747–76.

3. L. F. Berkman and S. L. Syme, "Social Networks, Host Resistance, and Mortality: A Nine-Year Follow-Up Study of Alameda County Residents," *American Journal of Epidemiology* 109, no. 2 (February 1979): 186–204; T. A. Glass et al., "Population-

Based Study of Social and Productive Activities as Predictors of Survival Among Elderly Americans," *British Medical Journal* 319, no. 7208 (August 21, 1999): 478–83; L. C. Giles et al., "Effect of Social Networks on Ten Year Survival in Very Old Australians: The Australian Longitudinal Study of Aging," *Journal of Epidemiology and Community Health* 59, no. 7 (July 2005): 574–79; J. S. House, C. Robbins, and H. L. Metzner, "The Association of Social Relationships and Activities with Mortality: Prospective Evidence from the Tecumseh Community Health Study," *American Journal of Epidemiology* 116, no. 1 (July 1982): 123–40.

4. P. Reynolds et al., "The Relationship Between Social Ties and Survival Among Black and White Breast Cancer Patients: National Cancer Institute Black/White Cancer Survival Study Group," *Cancer Epidemiology, Biomarkers, and Prevention: A Publication of the American Association for Cancer Research, Cosponsored by the American Society of Preventive Oncology* 3, no. 3 (April/May 1994): 253–59.

5. L. F. Berkman and S. L. Syme, "Social Networks, Host Resistance, and Mortality: A Nine-Year Follow-Up Study of Alameda County Residents," *American Journal of Epidemiology* 109, no. 2 (February 1979): 186–204; T. A. Glass et al., "Population-Based Study of Social and Productive Activities as Predictors of Survival Among Elderly Americans," *British Medical Journal* 319, no. 7208 (August 21, 1999): 478–83; S. Wolf and J. G. Bruhn, *The Power of Clan: The Influence of Human Relationships on Heart Disease* (Piscataway, NJ: Transaction Publishers, 1998); C. J. Holahan et al., "Late-Life Alcohol Consumption and Twenty-Year Mortality," *Alcoholism, Clinical and Experimental Research* 34, no. 11 (November 2010): 1961–71.

6. P. Reynolds et al., "The Relationship Between Social Ties and Survival Among Black and White Breast Cancer Patients: National Cancer Institute Black/White Cancer Survival Study Group," *Cancer Epidemiology, Biomarkers, and Prevention: A Publication of the American Association for Cancer Research, Cosponsored by the American Society of Preventive Oncology* 3, no. 3 (April/May 1994): 253–59; A. F. Chou et al., "Social Support and Survival in Young Women with Breast Carcinoma," *Psycho-oncology* 21, no. 2 (February 2012): 125–33; C. H. Kroenke et al., "Social Networks, Social Support, and Survival After Breast Cancer Diagnosis," *Journal of Clinical Oncology* 24, no. 7 (March 1, 2006): 1105–11; N. Waxler-Morrison et al., "Effects of Social Relationships on Survival for Women with Breast Cancer: A Prospective Study," *Social Science and Medicine* 33, no. 2 (1991): 177–83; K. L. Weihs et al., "Dependable Social Relationships Predict Overall Survival in Stages II and III Breast Carcinoma Patients," *Journal of Psychosomatic Research* 59, no. 5 (November 2005): 299–306; J. Holt-Lunstad, T. B. Smith, and J. B. Layton, "Social Relationships and Mortality Risk: A Meta-Analytic Review," *PLOS Medicine* 7, no. 7 (July 27, 2010): e1000316; A. Krongrad et al., "Marriage and Mortality in Prostate Cancer," *Journal of Urology* 156, no. 5 (November 1996): 1696–70; P. N. Butow, A. S. Coates, and S. M. Dunn, "Psychosocial Predictors of Survival in Metastatic Melanoma," *Journal of Clinical Oncology* 17, no. 7 (July 1999): 2256–63.

7. A. F. Chou et al., "Social Support and Survival in Young Women with Breast Carcinoma," *Psycho-oncology* 21, no. 2 (February 2012): 125–33.

8. M. Pinquart and P. R. Duberstein, "Associations of Social Networks with Cancer Mortality: A Meta-Analysis," *Critical Reviews in Oncology/Hematology* 75, no. 2 (August 2010): 122–37.

9. B. N. Uchino, J. T. Cacioppo, and J. K. Kiecolt-Glaser, "The Relationship Between Social Support and Physiological Processes: A Review with Emphasis on Underlying Mechanisms and Implications for Health," *Psychological Bulletin* 119, no. 3 (May 1996): 488–531; B. N. Uchino, "Social Support and Health: A Review of Physiological Processes Potentially Underlying Links to Disease Outcomes," *Journal of Behavioral Medicine* 29, no. 4 (August 2006): 377–87.

10. S. Dockray and A. Steptoe, "Positive Affect and Psychobiological Processes," *Neuroscience and Biobehavioral Reviews* 35, no. 1 (September 2010): 69–75; R. Ader, ed., *Psychoneuroimmunology,* 4th ed. (Burlington, MA: Elsevier Academic Press, 2011).

11. L. C. Giles et al., "Effect of Social Networks on Ten Year Survival in Very Old Australians: The Australian Longitudinal Study of Aging," *Journal of Epidemiology and Community Health* 59, no. 7 (July 2005): 574–79; J. S. House, C. Robbins, and H. L. Metzner, "The Association of Social Relationships and Activities with Mortality: Prospective Evidence from the Tecumseh Community Health Study," *American Journal of Epidemiology* 116, no. 1 (July 1982): 123–40.

12. A. Steptoe et al., "Social Isolation, Loneliness, and All-Cause Mortality in Older Men and Women," *Proceedings of the National Academy of Sciences of the United States of America* 110, no. 15 (April 9, 2013): 5797–801.

13. C. H. Kroenke et al., "Social Networks, Social Support, and Survival After Breast Cancer Diagnosis," *Journal of Clinical Oncology* 24, no. 7 (March 1, 2006): 1105–11.

14. J. T. Cacioppo et al., "Lonely Traits and Concomitant Physiological Processes: The MacArthur Social Neuroscience Studies," *International Journal of Psychophysiology* 35, nos. 2–3 (March 2000): 143–54.

15. B. N. Uchino, J. T. Cacioppo, and J. K. Kiecolt-Glaser, "The Relationship Between Social Support and Physiological Processes: A Review with Emphasis on Underlying Mechanisms and Implications for Health," *Psychological Bulletin* 119, no. 3 (May 1996): 488–531; J. K. Kiecolt-Glaser et al., "Psychosocial Modifiers of Immunocompetence in Medical Students," *Psychosomatic Medicine* 46, no. 1 (January/February 1984): 7–14; J. K. Kiecolt-Glaser et al., "Urinary Cortisol Levels, Cellular Immunocompetency, and Loneliness in Psychiatric Inpatients," *Psychosomatic Medicine* 46, no. 1 (January/February 1984): 15–23; S. D. Pressman et al., "Loneliness, Social Network Size, and Immune Response to Influenza Vaccination in College Freshmen," *Health Psychology* 24, no. 3 (May 2005): 297–306.

16. S. Dockray and A. Steptoe, "Positive Affect and Psychobiological Processes," *Neuroscience and Biobehavioral Reviews* 35, no. 1 (September 2010): 69–75; R. Ader, ed., *Psychoneuroimmunology,* 4th ed. (Burlington, MA: Elsevier Academic Press, 2011).

17. E. E. Benarroch, "Oxytocin and Vasopressin: Social Neuropeptides with Complex Neuromodulatory Functions," *Neurology* 80, no. 16 (April 16, 2013): 1521–28.

18. E. Friedmann and S. A. Thomas, "Pet Ownership, Social Support, and One-Year Survival After Acute Myocardial Infarction in the Cardiac Arrhythmia Suppression Trial (CAST)," *American Journal of Cardiology* 76, no. 17 (December 15, 1995): 1213–17; J. McNicholas et al., "Pet Ownership and Human Health: A Brief Review of Evidence and Issues," *British Medical Journal* 331, no. 7527 (November 26, 2005): 1252–54; R. W. Steele, "Should Immunocompromised Patients Have Pets?" *Ochsner Journal* 8, no. 3 (Fall 2008): 134–39; M. Müllersdorf et al., "Aspects of Health, Physical/Leisure Activities, Work and Socio-Demographics Associated with Pet Ownership in Sweden," *Scandinavian Journal of Public Health* 38, no. 1 (February 2010): 53–63; A. I. Qureshi et al., "Cat Ownership and the Risk of Fatal Cardiovascular Diseases: Results from the Second National Health and Nutrition Examination Study Mortality Follow-Up Study," *Journal of Vascular and Interventional Neurology* 2, no. 1 (January 2009): 132–35.

19. R. M. Nerem, M. J. Levesque, and J. F. Cornhill, "Social Environment as a Factor in Diet-Induced Atherosclerosis," *Science* 208, no. 4451 (June 27, 1980): 1475–76.

20. K. M. Grewen et al., "Effects of Partner Support on Resting Oxytocin, Cortisol, Norepinephrine, and Blood Pressure Before and After Warm Partner Contact," *Psychosomatic Medicine* 67, no. 4 (July/August 2005): 531–38.

CHAPTER 8: DEEPENING YOUR SPIRITUAL CONNECTION

1. National Sleep Foundation, "Sleep Aids and Insomnia," http://www.sleepfoundation.org/article/sleep-related-problems/sleep-aids-and-insomnia, accessed September 28, 2013; Anxiety and Depression Association of America, "Facts and Statistics," http://www.adaa.org/about-adaa/press-room/facts-statistics, accessed September 28, 2013.

2. G. A. Tooley et al., "Acute Increases in Night-time Plasma Melatonin Levels Following a Period of Meditation," *Biological Psychology* 53, no. 1 (May 2000): 69–78.

3. F. D. Ganz, "Sleep and Immune Function," *Critical Care Nurse* 32, no. 2 (April 2012): e19–25.

4. L. Tamarkin et al., "Decreased Nocturnal Plasma Melatonin Peak in Patients with Estrogen Receptor Positive Breast Cancer," *Science* 216, no. 4549 (May 28, 1982): 1003–5; S. Davis and D. K. Mirick, "Circadian Disruption, Shift Work and the Risk of Cancer: A Summary of the Evidence and Studies in Seattle," *Cancer Causes and Control* 17, no. 4 (May 2006): 539–45.

5. B. K. Hölzel et al., "Mindfulness Practice Leads to Increases in Regional Brain Gray Matter Density," *Psychiatry Research* 191, no. 1 (January 30, 2011): 36–43.

6. D. N. Khansari, A. J. Murgo, and R. E. Faith, "Effects of Stress on the Immune System," *Immunology Today* 11, no. 5 (May 1990): 170–75; S. B. Pruett, "Stress and the Immune System," *Pathophysiology* 9, no. 3 (May 2003): 133–53; S. C. Segerstrom and G. E. Miller, "Psychological Stress and the Human Immune System: A

Meta-Analytic Study of Thirty Years of Inquiry," *Psychological Bulletin* 130, no. 4 (July 2004): 601–30.

7. R. J. Davidson et al., "Alterations in Brain and Immune Function Produced by Mindfulness Meditation," *Psychosomatic Medicine* 65, no. 4 (July/August 2003): 564–70.

8. T. L. Jacobs et al., "Intensive Meditation Training, Immune Cell Telomerase Activity, and Psychological Mediators," *Psychoneuroendocrinology* 36, no. 5 (June 2011): 664–81.

9. J. A. Dusek et al., "Genomic Counter-Stress Changes Induced by the Relaxation Response," *PLOS ONE* 3, no. 7 (2008): e2576.

CHAPTER 9: HAVING STRONG REASONS FOR LIVING

1. S. Greer, T. Morris, and K. W. Pettingale, "Psychological Response to Breast Cancer: Effect on Outcome," *The Lancet* 2, no. 8146 (October 13, 1979): 785–87.

2. R. H. Osborne et al., "Immune Function and Adjustment Style: Do They Predict Survival in Breast Cancer?" *Psycho-oncology* 13, no. 3 (March 2004): 199–210; P. N. Butow, A. S. Coates, and S. M. Dunn, "Psychosocial Predictors of Survival in Metastatic Melanoma," *Journal of Clinical Oncology* 17, no. 7 (July 1999): 2256–63; P. N. Butow, A. S. Coates, and S. M. Dunn, "Psychosocial Predictors of Survival: Metastatic Breast Cancer," *Annals of Oncology: Official Journal of the European Society for Medical Oncology* 11, no. 4 (April 2000): 469–74.

3. M. S. Vos et al., "Denial and Physical Outcomes in Lung Cancer Patients: A Longitudinal Study," *Lung Cancer* 67, no. 2 (February 2010): 237–43.

4. M. Watson et al., "Influence of Psychological Response on Survival in Breast Cancer: A Population-Based Cohort Study," *The Lancet* 354, no. 9187 (October 16, 1999): 1331–36; M. Pinquart and P. R. Duberstein, "Depression and Cancer Mortality: A Meta-Analysis," *Psychological Medicine* 40, no. 11 (November 2010): 1797–810; W. F. Pirl et al., "Depression and Survival in Metastatic Non-Small-Cell Lung Cancer: Effects of Early Palliative Care," *Journal of Clinical Oncology* 30, no. 12 (April 20, 2012): 1310–15; H. Faller and M. Schmidt, "Prognostic Value of Depressive Coping and Depression in Survival of Lung Cancer Patients," *Psycho-oncology* 13, no. 5 (May 2004): 359–63; J. S. Goodwin, D. D. Zhang, and G. V. Ostir, "Effect of Depression on Diagnosis, Treatment, and Survival of Older Women with Breast Cancer," *Journal of the American Geriatrics Society* 52, no. 1 (January 2004): 106–11.

5. H. Yu et al., "Depression and Survival in Chinese Patients with Gastric Cancer: A Prospective Study," *Asian Pacific Journal of Cancer Prevention* 13, no. 1 (2012): 391–94; M. Johansson, A. Rydén, and C. Finizia, "Mental Adjustment to Cancer and Its Relation to Anxiety, Depression, HRQL, and Survival in Patients with Laryngeal Cancer: A Longitudinal Study," *BMC Cancer* 11 (June 30, 2011): 283; K. E. Lazure et al., "Association Between Depression and Survival or Disease Recurrence in Patients with Head and Neck Cancer Enrolled in a Depression Prevention Trial," *Head and Neck* 31, no. 7 (July 2009): 888–92.

6. M. Petticrew, R. Bell, and D. Hunter, "Influence of Psychological Coping on Survival and Recurrence in People with Cancer: Systematic Review," *British Medical
Journal* 325, no. 7372 (November 9, 2002): 1066.

7. A. J. Cunningham and K. Watson, "How Psychological Therapy May Prolong Survival in Cancer Patients: New Evidence and a Simple Theory," *Integrative Cancer
Therapies* 3, no. 3 (September 2004): 214–29; R. Huebscher, "Spontaneous Remission of Cancer: An Example of Health Promotion," *Nurse Practitioner Forum* 3, no.
4 (December 1992): 228–35.

8. M. Watson et al., "Influence of Psychological Response on Breast Cancer Survival:
Ten-Year Follow-Up of a Population-Based Cohort," *European Journal of Cancer* 41,
no. 12 (August 2005): 1710–14.

9. J. Giese-Davis et al., "Decrease in Depression Symptoms Is Associated with Longer
Survival in Patients with Metastatic Breast Cancer: A Secondary Analysis," *Journal
of Clinical Oncology* 29, no. 4 (February 1, 2011): 413–20.

10. H. Karppinen et al., "Will-to-Live and Survival in a Ten-Year Follow-Up Among
Older People," *Age and Ageing* 41, no. 6 (November 2012): 789–94.

CONCLUSION

1. N. Howlader et al., *SEER Cancer Statistics Review, 1975–2009.* (Bethesda, MD:
National Cancer Institute.) Based on November 2011 SEER data submission.

2. Bryan Walsh, "Sixty Years After Man First Climbed Everest, the Mountain
Is a Mess," *Time Science and Space* online, May 29, 2013, http://science.time
.com/2013/05/29/60-years-after-man-first-climbed-everest-the-mountain-is-a-
mess/.

INDEX

ABOUT THE AUTHOR

KELLY TURNER, PH.D., is a researcher, author, and lecturer in the field of integrative oncology and the founder of the Radical Remission Project. Her specialized research focus is the Radical Remission of cancer, which is a remission that occurs either in the absence of Western medicine, or after Western medicine has failed to achieve remission. Dr. Turner's interest in complementary medicine began when she received her B.A. from Harvard University, and it later became the sole focus of her Ph.D. at the University of California, Berkeley. Her dissertation research included a year-long trip around the world, for which she traveled to ten different countries to interview fifty alternative healers and twenty Radical Remission cancer survivors about their healing techniques. Since then, her ongoing research has led her to analyze over one thousand cases of Radical Remission and to found the Radical Remission Project, an interactive website and database of Radical Remission cases (see www.RadicalRemission.com). When she's not studying or lecturing about Radical Remission, you will likely find her snuggling up with her family or writing screenplays. For more information on Dr. Turner, visit www.DrKellyTurner.com.

SCAN THIS CODE
WITH YOUR SMARTPHONE TO BE LINKED TO THE BONUS MATERIALS FOR

RADICAL REMISSION

on the Elixir website,
where you can also find information about other
healthy living books and related materials.

YOU CAN ALSO TEXT
REMISSION to READIT (732348)

to be sent a link to the Elixir website.